MfBackhouse

6.50

PAEDIATRIC EMERGENCIES

A Houseman's Pocketbook

Christopher Bacon, M.R.C.P.

LONDON
WILLIAM HEINEMANN MEDICAL BOOKS

First published 1982

ISBN 0-433-01051-7

Computer typesetting by Method Limited,
8 The Broadway, Woodford Green, Essex,
and printed in Great Britain by Redwood Burn Limited,
Trowbridge Wiltshire

Introduction

These notes were originally compiled for quick reference on the ward, and have proved their value for paediatric house staff in the prompt diagnosis and treatment of sick children at times when experienced advice is not immediately at hand. There are chapters covering most of the common acute illnesses of childhood, and the advice given is based on well-established practices and does not required sophisticated facilities. The text is deliberately terse and didactic: there is no room for discussion or references, nor the reminder, which might appear on every page, that for a sick child and his family a sympathetic approach is always an essential part of management. There is also a chapter containing notes on practical procedures, and an appendix outlining various data such as fluid requirements and drug dosages.

Care of the sick newborn should be in specialist hands, but sometimes a junior paediatrician has to cover a maternity unit and may be faced with an unexpected emergency, so a chapter on the commoner neonatal problems is included, but it is very elementary and condensed, and offers little more than 'first aid' until more expert care is available.

Acknowledgements

I should like to thank many colleagues and friends in Newcastle for their generous help in the compilation of these notes, and Shirley Holmes who patiently typed several drafts of the manuscript.

Contents

1 *Respiratory System*

ACUTE STRIDOR

Clinical

Stridor is an **inspiratory** sound caused by partial obstruction of the upper airway, and when severe is accompanied by soft tissue recession and respiratory distress.

Diagnosis

1. The main causes are

   (i) viral laryngitis ('croup')
   (ii) epiglottitis
   (iii) foreign body (p. 8)

(Also measles, diphtheria, allergic oedema, retropharyngeal abscess, hypocalcaemia.)

2. Distinction between croup and epiglottitis is very important because croup is common but not usually serious, while epiglottitis is less common but always dangerous.
3. Distinctive features are outlined in Table 1.1.

Management

Diagnosis uncertain

1. If you suspect epiglottitis, but cannot easily see the epiglottis, do not poke about in the back of the throat as this may precipitate obstruction. Arrange urgent laryngoscopy in theatre.
2. Take blood for culture and w.b.c.
3. Get lateral x-ray of neck, which may show swollen epiglottis

Table 1.1. Distinctive features of viral laryngitis and epiglottitis

	Viral laryngitis	*Epiglottitis*
Typical age	3 months – 3 years	18 months – 7 years
Cause	Several respiratory viruses, especially para-influenza	*Haemophilus influenzae* (type B)
Usual associated features	Sometimes history of previous attacks; coryza; barking cough; hoarseness	Sore throat; cervical adenopathy; drooling; muffled voice
Systemic illness	Usually slight or moderate	Usually severe, with high fever
Progression	Usually gradual	Often rapid, with abrupt onset of severe obstruction
Epiglottis (if visible)	Normal or mildly inflamed	Swollen and bright red
White blood count	Variable; often normal	Usually polymorph leucocytosis

(make sure child is accompanied by doctor or competent nurse while in x-ray department).

4. If there is no fever or other evidence of infection, suspect a foreign body.

Epiglottitis

1. **Arrange for urgent intubation.** Ideally this should be done by an anaesthetist in theatre with all prepared for tracheostomy in case intubation fails. In extreme emergency try intubation yourself (p. 168).

2. Put up a drip and give
   - (i) fluid requirements
   - (ii) i.v. chloramphenicol (preferable to ampicillin in this situation).

Viral laryngitis

1. Give humidified oxygen.
2. Keep child as calm as possible, preferably with his mother beside him.
3. If very agitated, and not exhausted and not in respiratory failure, give mild sedation (e.g. trimeprazine).
4. If obstruction severe or deteriorating, or if evidence of respiratory failure (p. 11), arrange urgent intubation (as for epiglottitis, above).

Foreign body

See p. 8.

ASTHMATIC ATTACKS

Clinical

The wheeze of asthma comes from the lower airways and is predominantly **expiratory.** It is often accompanied by rhonchi, soft tissue recession and respiratory distress. In small children the attack is often preceded by coryza and, for the purpose of this section, 'wheezy bronchitis' is regarded as the same as asthma.

Diagnosis

1. Always consider possibility of aspirated foreign body (p. 8), especially in a child who has not wheezed before.

2. If diagnosis in doubt or unusual clinical features get chest x-ray looking for

(i) pneumothorax (p. 9)
(ii) collapse/consolidation
(iii) signs of aspirated foreign body.

Management

1. If any evidence of hypoxia, give humidified 100% **oxygen**.
2. Nurse child propped at about 45°.
3. Give **corticosteroids** (corticosteroids do no harm when given in occasional short courses, and should be started straight away because they take a few hours to work fully — (for dosages, see p. 186):

(i) if attack moderately severe give oral prednisolone, reducing as improvement proceeds
(ii) if more severe give i.v. hydrocortisone on admission and 2 - 4 hourly until improvement begins, then switch to oral prednisolone.

4. Give **bronchodilators** (for dosages see p. 186):

(i) find out what has been given before admission so as to avoid overdosage
(ii) whenever possible give nebulised salbutamol which is quickest and safest, and can be repeated 3 hourly until attack subsides (if child will not tolerate mask or mouth-piece ask his mother to hold it close to his mouth and give extra solution)
(iii) if attack very severe give i.v. aminophylline (slow loading bolus followed by infusion: too rapid administration can be dangerous) as well as nebulised salbutamol
(iv) if you cannot get drip up and nebuliser not available give salbutamol i.m. or s.c.

5. Sedate with your calmness, not with drugs.
6. If attack very severe put up a drip

   (i) to ensure hydration
   (ii) for drugs.

7. If there is collapse/consolidation give cotrimoxazole.
8. If condition severe or deteriorating do blood gases, and see *Respiratory Failure* (p. 11). Do not be misled by child whose wheeze diminishes as he gets more exhausted.
9. If there is rapid deterioration at any time repeat chest x-ray in case pneumothorax has developed.
10. If child <12 months old, treat as for bronchiolitis.

BRONCHIOLITIS

Clinical

Bronchiolitis occurs mainly in winter epidemics of respiratory syncytial virus and affects babies up to 2 years old. Others in the family may have a cold, and the baby's illness starts as coryza, progressing to respiratory distress, with cough, tachypnoea, wheezing, scattered crepitations and soft tissue recession.

Diagnosis

1. The main differential diagnoses are pneumonia (p. 6) or heart failure (p. 16).
2. Chest x-ray in bronchiolitis shows

   (i) usually over-inflation (more than 9 posterior rib origins above diaphragm on PA film)
   (ii) sometimes small areas of shadowing caused by atelectasis.

3. White cell count is variable; polymorph leucocytosis suggests bacterial infection.

Management

1. Nurse baby propped at 45°.
2. Keep him warm (in incubator if small baby with severe illness).
3. Give humidified oxygen (p. 12).
4. If secretions copious, gently suck out oro- and naso-pharynx 1 - 2 hourly with a fine catheter.
5. Fluids
   (i) if condition moderate, feed by naso-gastric tube 2 hourly
   (ii) if severe, put up a drip and hydrate i.v.
6. If condition severe or deteriorating do blood gases and see *Respiratory Failure* (p. 11).
7. Do not give physiotherapy, which is exhausting and probably useless.
8. The following drugs are not helpful, and may sometimes be harmful:

   Bronchodilators
   Cortiscosteroids
   Sedatives
   Digoxin (unless heart abnormal)

9. If possibility of pneumonia give antibiotics (p. 8).

PNEUMONIA

(for pneumonia in neonates see p. 135)

Clinical

Pneumonia is often preceded by upper respiratory infection, and typical features are cough, tachypnoea, flushed face, flaring alae nasi, expiratory grunt, bronchial breathing and crepitations.

There is usually high fever (though infants may sometimes be hypothermic).

Diagnosis

1. In children pneumonia may sometimes present as

Meningism	Delirium
Abdominal pain	Collapse

2. In babies under 2 years the main differential diagnoses are bronchiolitis (p. 5) or heart failure (p. 16).
3. Consolidation on chest x-ray is diagnostic.
4. There is usually marked polymorph leucocytosis, except when infection is not bacterial.

Management

1. Get chest x-ray (PA and lateral).
2. Take blood for

w.b.c.	Mycoplasma and viral antibodies
Culture	

3. If condition severe or deteriorating do blood gases and see *Respiratory Failure* (p. 11).
4. Try to get sputum or a cough swab for bacterial culture, and take swabs for viral studies.
5. Ensure adequate hydration, by drip if necessary.
6. Consider physiotherapy.
7. Give paracetamol to relieve pain and reduce fever.
8. Start antibiotics, parenterally for at least 48 hours, as shown in Table 1.2.

Table 1.2 Use of antibiotics for child with pneumonia

Age	*Most likely organism*	*Antibiotic*
< 1 month (see p. 135)		
1 month – 2 years	*Staph. aureus* pneumococcus	benzyl penicillin + flucloxacillin
> 2 years	pneumococcus	benzyl penicillin
Special cases		
Child with cystic fibrosis	*Staph. aureus* *Pseudomonas*	flucloxacillin + carbenicillin
Child with asthma	various	cotrimoxazole
Chest x-ray shows pneumatocoeles or abscesses	*Staph. aureus*	flucloxacillin

ASPIRATED FOREIGN BODY

Clinical

Foreign bodies are most commonly aspirated by children aged 2 months to 4 years, and the typical object is a peanut or small bead. There is not always a history of choking, and symptoms may sometimes not start for several days.

Diagnosis

1. If foreign body is in larynx or trachea, symptoms may resemble croup, with cough and stridor.
2. If foreign body is in bronchus, symptoms may resemble asthma, with dyspnoea and wheeze.

3. Stridor and wheeze may be

   (i) inspiratory more than expiratory
   (ii) intermittent, variable and of unusual tone
   (iii) unilateral.

4. Be particularly suspicious of

   (i) stridor in a child without fever or respiratory infection
   (ii) wheezing in a child without previous attacks
   (iii) pneumonia of a lower lobe not responding to treatment.

Management

1. Get x-rays of neck (PA and lateral) or chest (PA and lateral, inspiration and expiration) looking for

   (i) opaque foreign body
   (ii) overinflation of lung or lobe on expiratory film (obstructive emphysema)
   (iii) partial or complete collapse of lung or part of it.

2. If any suspicion, clinically or on x-ray, arrange early laryngoscopy or bronchoscopy.

PNEUMOTHORAX

(for pneumothorax in neonates see p. 135)

General

1. Pneumothorax in children usually occurs as a complication of

Asthma
Bronchiolitis
Pneumonia (especially staphylococcal)
Trauma
Positive pressure respiration

2. Spontaneous pneumothorax is rare, but may occur in older children.

Diagnosis

1. Typical features are

   (i) sudden deterioration in previous illness
   (ii) chest pain of sudden onset
   (iii) dyspnoea, tachypnoea, cyanosis (if severe)
   (iv) hyper-resonance and diminished breath sounds over part of chest.

2. Chest x-ray (inspiratory and expiratory) is diagnostic.

Management

1. Usually a pneumothorax can be left to absorb by itself, but it should be drained urgently if

   (i) it is under tension
   (ii) it is seriously aggravating the severity of underlying illness.

2. Tension may be indicated by

   (i) deviation of trachea and displacement of apex beat (mark initial position)
   (ii) rising pulse and increasing dyspnoea.

3. If in doubt repeat chest x-ray.
4. If any suggestion of hypoxia give 100% oxygen.
5. For technique of chest drainage, see p. 166.

RESPIRATORY FAILURE

(for respiratory failure in neonates, see p. 133)

General

Respiratory failure in children may result from:

Status asthmaticus
Pneumonia
Bronchiolitis
Upper respiratory obstruction

Decreased respiratory effort due to poisoning, encephalitis, head injury or paralysis

Diagnosis

1. Respiratory failure is difficult to assess by clinical features alone so always do blood gases.

2. **Moderate failure** may be accompanied by

(i) restlessness and irritability
(ii) inability to talk, eat or sleep
(iii) rising pulse
(iv) rising respiratory rate
(v) increasing soft tissue retraction
(vi) pulsus paradoxus

(iv)–(vi): (not when cause is decreased respiratory effort)

3. **Severe failure** may be accompanied by

(i) central cyanosis, which indicates $P_{O_2} <$ c. 7kPa (look at tongue, not periphery; allow for anaemia when cyanosis appears later, and for polycythaemia when it appears earlier)
(ii) peripheral vasoconstriction (hypoxia) or peripheral vasodilatation (hypercapnia)
(iii) decrease in air entry, which may cause misleading diminution in stridor or wheeze
(iv) irregular respiration or periods of apnoea

(v) hypotonia and exhaustion
(vi) falling level of consciousness, or convulsions.

Management

1. Do blood gases (see below) as a base-line and repeat at intervals according to initial result and clinical progress (for technique, see p. 153).

2. Treat the cause. If the cause is upper respiratory obstruction arrange urgent intubation or tracheostomy.

3. If respiratory failure severe or deteriorating consult anaethetist at once about assisted ventilation.

4. If any evidence of hypoxia give oxygen in concentration high enough to relieve it, 100% if necessary. Oxygen therapy in acute respiratory failure in children does not usually reduce the respiratory drive and a high P_{O_2} carries little risk (except in neonates, p. 134). Routes with their maximum oxygen concentrations are as follows

in an incubator	(c. 85%)
with a head box	(c. 90%)
in a tent	(c. 75%)
by mask	(100%)
by nasal cannulae	(c. 95%)

5. Put up a drip and hydrate i.v.

6. If pH <7.25 correct with slow infusion of sodium bicarbonate (see formula on p. 77).

Blood gases

1. Always interpret blood gas figures in conjunction with the clinical state. Change is more important than a single reading.

2. **P_{CO_2}**

(i) is usually the most helpful
(ii) does not vary much with ambient oxygen concentration

(iii) may fall at first in some conditions (e.g. asthma) due to hyperventilation
(iv) if rising above normal usually indicates serious respiratory failure
(v) can be assessed accurately from arterial or capillary blood, and approximately from mixed venous blood.

3. ***P_{O_2}***

(i) varies markedly with ambient oxygen concentration
(ii) may be decreased because of either hypoventilation or mismatch
(iii) can be assessed accurately from arterial blood, approximately from capillary blood, and not at all from venous blood.

4. As a rough guide respiratory failure can usually be described as

present when

$P_{CO_2} > 6.5$ kPa
and/or
$P_{O_2} < 9$ kPa in air

severe when

$P_{CO_2} > 8.5$ kPa
and/or
$P_{O_2} < 5$ kPa in air
or
$P_{O_2} < 8.0$ kPa in 50% oxygen

(for normal values see p. 184).

OTITIS MEDIA

General

1. Otitis media is very common in small children. Although not life-threatening it may have serious sequelae if not treated promptly.

2. Infection may be viral or bacterial. Since the two cannot easily be distinguished and the former may lead to the latter, it is best to treat all otitis media (unless trivial) as bacterial.

Clinical

1. Otitis media usually accompanies or follows an upper respiratory infection, and tends to recur in the same child.
2. It may present as

(i) pulling the ears, or shaking the head
(ii) screaming or misery
(iii) fever, or a febrile convulsion
(iv) meningism
(v) poor feeding or vomiting (and sometimes diarrhoea).

3. A 'discharge' is more often due to melted wax than suppuration.
4. Always examine the ear drums of any ill child. Make sure a small child is held properly (sitting on mother's or nurse's knee sideways on, with one of her hands holding his head to her chest, and the other holding his trunk and arms).
5. If wax at first obscures the drum, try and peer round it. If this is not possible, remove some of the wax *very cautiously*, with the child held firmly, using a tuft of cotton wool on a loop of fine flexible wire (e.g. 10 amp fuse wire).

Management

1. Take swabs from

(i) nose and throat (though these may be irrelevant)
(ii) if drum has burst, from discharge.

2. If drums are more than minimally inflamed, treat with

(i) antibiotics
(ii) decongestants.

Table 1.3 Use of antibiotics for child with otitis media

	Organism	*Antibiotic* (for doses, see p. 185)
Children under 3 years old	*Haemophilus* pneumococcus	cotrimoxazole or amoxycillin
Older children	pneumococcus *Streptococcus*	penicillin
Chronic suppurative otitis	various	cotrimoxazole initially, then according to culture result

3. Most likely bacteria and appropriate antibiotics are shown in Table 1.3.

4. Antibiotics should be given for at least 10 days. Start i.m. for 1-3 days if

(i) drums are bulging
(ii) mastoid process is tender
(iii) child is at risk of febrile convulsion
(iv) child is in pain.

5. Decongestants may help open Eustachian tubes, especially in smaller children, and can be given

(i) by mouth (e.g. *Triominic, Actifed*)
(ii) as nose drops (e.g. 0.5% ephedrine).

6. Myringotomy, which should be done only by an ENT surgeon, is seldom required in acute otitis unless

(i) drums seems likely to burst
(ii) pain is severe and prolonged.

2 *Cardiovascular System*

HEART FAILURE

General

Heart failure in children most commonly occurs in infancy as a result of congenital heart disease, where early diagnosis and treatment may be vital. It may occasionally occur in older children from conditions such as myocarditis or severe anaemia.

Diagnosis

1. In older children the clinical features are as in adults.
2. Features of heart failure in infants are

   (i) dyspnoea and exhaustion on feeding (often the earliest symptom noted by the mother)
   (ii) fast and laboured breathing, sometimes with wheezing and recession
   (iii) tachycardia, with gallop rhythm
   (iv) sweating
   (v) poor peripheral circulation
   (vi) fluid retention, noticeable by excess weight gain and oedema round the eyes and on dorsa of feet
   (vii) enlarging liver
   (viii) large heart on chest x-ray

3. Distinguish from bronchiolitis (p. 5) or pneumonia (p. 6), which have several features in common.

Management

1. Consult a cardiologist *early* in case there is a lesion needing urgent correction.

2. Nurse propped in a chair or on a slope, or in a tilted incubator.

3. If there is hypoxia or poor peripheral circulation give 100% oxygen.

4. Do the following investigations:

Chest x-ray	Arterial gases (if central cyanosis in doubt)
ECG	
Hb, electrolytes and urea	

5. Feed as follows:

(i) two hourly, so as to give daily need in small amounts
(ii) low sodium milk (e.g. expressed breast milk, SMA *Gold Cap*, Cow and Gate *Premium*, Ostermilk *Complete*)
(iii) by nasogastric tube (left *in situ*).

6. Drugs:

(i) digoxin in full dose (p. 186)
(ii) frusemide, with K^+ supplements, if failure severe
(iii) mild sedation if restless.

7. If anaemic, transfuse slowly (e.g. 30 ml/h) using packed cells and frusemide cover.

8. Correct severe acidosis (p. 77), which impairs myocardial function, but beware of sodium overload.

9. Monitor pulse, respiration rate and fluid balance, and weigh daily.

SHOCK

General

Shock is used here to describe any state in which the circulation is so impaired that there is a risk of inadequate perfusion of vital organs. In small children shock occurs more rapidly and in a wider range of conditions than in adults.

Diagnosis

1. The typical features are

    (i) pallor and peripheral cyanosis (and sometimes mottled skin in babies)
    (ii) cold extremities, sometimes clammy with sweat
    (iii) rapid feeble pulse, collapsed veins, and blood pressure low or unrecordable
    (iv) acidotic respiration

2. The main causes are

    (i) severe infection, such as
        septicaemia (p. 33)
        pneumonia (p. 6)
        peritonitis (p. 59)
    (ii) hypovolaemia, resulting from
        gastro-enteritis (p. 63)
        haemorrhage (p. 28)
        diabetic ketosis (p. 68)
        severe burns (p. 103)
    (iii) poisoning (p. 79)
    (iv) heart failure (p. 16)
    (v) intracranial haemorrhage (p. 43)
    (vi) anaphylaxis.

Management

1. Minimise **cerebral hypoxia**

    (i) give 100% oxygen by mask
    (ii) tilt head down.

2. Restore circulating **blood volume** (unless cause of shock is heart failure):

(i) get a drip up (if no success after two attempts do a cut-down – p. 157).
(ii) in an haemorrhage give highest fluid available on list below until matched blood arrives:

unmatched blood of same group
group O Rh –ve blood
plasma
dextran (take blood for cross-match first)
0.9% saline

(iii) in other conditions run in plasma 30 ml/kg fast, then modify as appropriate.

3. Take blood for

Hb and w.b.c	Glucose
Electrolytes and urea	Drug assay
Culture	(if poisoning possible).
Group and cross-match	

4. Treat the cause vigorously

(i) if cause known, see under relevant heading
(ii) if anaphylaxis give i.v. chlorpheniramine and hydrocortisone
(iii) if no cause evident, treat as for septicaemia (p. 33).

5. Monitor pulse, blood pressure and urine output.

6. If serum bicarbonate <10 mmol/l correct with i.v. bicarbonate (p. 77).

7. If shock does not respond to infusion of plasma and blood and to correction of acidosis

(i) put up a CVP line and run in more blood until CVP pressure reads +5 cm H_2O
(ii) give hydrocortisone i.v.
(iii) consider use of phenoxybenzamine to improve tissue perfusion (do *not* do this unless you have a CVP line up because it may cause a rapid drop in blood pressure).

CARDIAC DYSRHYTHMIAS

General

Cardiac dysrhythmias are uncommon in children. They may be idiopathic or secondary.

Diagnosis

1. The main idiopathic dysrhythmias are

(i) heart block
(ii) paroxysmal atrial tachycardia (PAT).

2. Secondary dysrhythmias may occur in association with

(i) congenital heart disease or after cardiac surgery
(ii) myocarditis or toxaemia
(iii) biochemical disturbance (e.g. acidosis, hypokalaemia)
(iv) poisoning (e.g. digoxin, tricyclics).

3. For identification of dysrhythmias consult a specialist textbook.

Management

1. Get a 12-lead ECG with rhythm strips on leads II and V1, and keep the child on a cardiac monitor.

2. Usually there is time to get a cardiologist's advice, but you should treat urgently if there is

(i) inadequate cerebral circulation (causing syncope)
(ii) inadequate coronary perfusion (causing angina)
(iii) heart failure.

3. If there is inadequate cerebral circulation

(i) keep child lying with head down
(ii) give 100% oxygen
(iii) consider cardiac massage (p. 25).

4. If there is heart failure, treat as on p. 16.
5. If there is no clear explanation for dysrhythmia

   (i) investigate possibility of poisoning.
   (ii) check serum potassium and bicarbonate.

Notes on individual dysrhythmias

Sinus arrhythmia

Often pronounced in children. Harmless.

Sinus bradycardia

If causing symptoms give atropine 0.2 - 0.6 mg i.v.

Sinus tachycardia

1. May be extreme during fever, etc (e.g. 160/min in an older child, 200/min in an infant).
2. Not harmful and requires no treatment in itself, but may be a sign of serious illness (e.g. heart failure, septicaemia).
3. An ECG may be necessary to distinguish from PAT, especially in an infant: either rhythm may accompany heart failure, one the cause, the other the effect.

Paroxysmal atrial tachycardia (PAT)

1. Rate usually 160-300/min. The commonest tachyarrhythmia in children.
2. May be associated with pre-excitation (Wolff-Parkinson-White).
3. PAT in infants may present as heart failure. Older children are usually aware of the onset.
4. In older children it may sometimes be stopped by vagal excitation:

   (i) ice-cream eaten quickly or ice-cold water gulped down

(ii) Valsalva manoeuvre
(iii) massage of carotid sinus (one at a time for 15 secs)
(iv) pressure on eye-ball
(v) induced vomiting.

5. If 4 does not work proceed to one of the following (for dosages see p. 186):

(i) i.m. digoxin
(ii) i.v. propranolol
(iii) DC shock (see p. 23)

Ventricular tachycardia

1. Rare except in myocarditis or intoxication.
2. Treat by (for dosages see p. 186)

(i) i.v. lignocaine
(ii) i.v. phenytoin
(iii) DC shock.

Ventricular fibrillation

1. See *Cardiac arrest* (p. 24)
2. Treat by DC shock immediately (see p. 23). The sooner you do it the greater the chance of success.

Digitalis poisoning

1. Worse if accompanied by hypokalaemia.
2. Causes a variety of dysrhythmias, among the most dangerous being

(i) atrial tachycardia with block
(ii) ventricular tachycardia.

3. If ingestion of digoxin <8 hours beforehand empty stomach (p. 80).
4. Take blood for

(i) electrolytes and urea
(ii) digitalis level.

5. If dysrhythmia life-threatening, put up a drip and start infusing potassium chloride in 5% dextrose at rate of 0.25 mmol/kg/h, modifying according to serum potassium levels.

6. Give either (for dosages see p. 186):

(i) i.v. phenytoin
(ii) i.v. propranolol.

7. Do not use DC shock unless ventricular fibrillation develops.

8. Stop digoxin and any diuretic that causes loss of potassium.

Complete heart block

Usually asymptomatic in children, but if causing heart failure or syncope

(i) consult cardiologist with a view to inserting pacemaker
(ii) meanwhile infuse isoprenalin *slowly* (e.g. 0.4 mg in 500 ml 5% dextrose), adjusting drip rate so as to speed heart enough without causing ectopic beats.

DC shock

1. Essential in ventricular fibrillation and often helpful in tachycardia (except those due to digitalis).

2. If possible avoid DC shock when digitalis has been given in the past 24 hours.

3. Unless child is unconscious do under general anaesthetic or heavy sedation.

4. Put one plate at left sternal border and the other behind left scapula.

5. Be careful not to get jelly smeared between the plates, which may cause dangerous arcing.

6. In supraventricular tachycardia synchronise the shock with the *R* wave.

7. Suitable initial charges are

(i) infant: 5 - 20 J
(ii) toddler: 20 - 100 J
(iii) older child: 100 - 200 J.

In fibrillation, if first shock ineffective double the charge.

CARDIAC ARREST

General

1. Cardiac arrest in children is often due to a temporary condition so resuscitation must always be attempted.
2. Always familiarise yourself thoroughly with resuscitation equipment on your wards, and ask nurses to do a practice drill with you.
3. If a child with a serious handicap develops a critical illness, establish in advance what the policy is about resuscitation.
4. A child can be kept alive for a long time by efficient mouth-to-mouth ventilation and cardiac massage. If you are the only doctor present concentrate on these two essentials until help arrives, and do not be diverted by drips and ECGs, which are less vital. Delegate tasks to nurses.

Diagnosis

1. Treat as for cardiac arrest any child who is cyanosed and has an impalpable apex beat and impalpable femoral and carotid pulses.
2. Do not spend more than a few moments listening with a stethoscope: cerebral necrosis begins within 2 min of cardiac arrest.
3. Apnoea is not always immediately accompanied by cardiac

arrest, so check the heart beat of an apnoeic child before beginning massage.

4. Cardiac massage is required not only for fibrillation and asystole, but also for rhythms giving inadequate circulation, such as extreme bradycardia or ventricular tachycardia.

Management

1. Send for:

- Anaesthetist (or cardiac arrest team
- Sucker
- Oxygen
- Bag and mask, and airways of various sizes
- Intubation equipment
- Drip set, 8.4% $NaHCO_3$ and 5% dextrose
- Cardiac monitor and defibrillator

2. Try a sharp blow to the praecordium (sometimes provokes a heart beat from asystole).

3. Unless child is small (e.g. <5 years) put him on floor with feet elevated.

4. Start **cardiac massage**

   (i) **in infants**, with finger tips only over *mid*-sternum, at 100 beats/min
   (ii) **in larger children** with heel of hand, over lower third of sternum, at 80 beats/min
   (iii) press strongly enough to produce a palpable femoral pulse
   (iv) do not press too low, especially in infants, or you may damage the liver.

5. Clear the airway

   (i) remove vomit and secretions by suction (or fingers if no sucker available)

(ii) elevate the chin
(iii) insert an airway.

6. Start **artificial respiration** immediately by the best means available — do not wait for equipment to arrive:

(i) mouth-to-mouth (p. 164)
(ii) bag and mask } with 100% oxygen
(iii) endotracheal intubation (p. 168) } with 100% oxygen

7. Put up a **drip** and run in

(i) 8.4% $NaHCO_3$, 1 ml/kg immediately, and repeat every 5 min while arrest continues
(ii) 5% dextrose at 30 ml/h in between.

8. Set up cardiac monitor and defibrillator. Stop cardiac massage and watch the pattern for not more than 10 sec at a time:

(i) if ventricular fibrillation, use DC shock immediately (see p. 000)
(ii) if asystole, try and induce fibrillation
(iii) if in doubt, try DC shock anyway.

9. To **induce fibrillation** give

(i) adrenalin 1/10 000 2 - 5 ml
(ii) calcium gluconate 10% 5 ml

either i.v. if you have a good drip, or by intracardiac injection (insert needle into 4th left interspace just below and medial to nipple — aim for spine — advance needle, frequently drawing back on syringe till free flow of blood indicates penetration of heart chamber — inject drugs).

10. Take arterial blood for gas estimation (or from heart if giving intracardiac injection), and adjust $NaHCO_3$ accordingly.

11. Continue attempts at resuscitation for at least 30 min.

12. Expect dysrhythmias once heart beat restarts and treat as on p.20.

13. If severe cerebral hypoxia has occurred, give dexamethasone.

14. Transfer child to intensive therapy unit in case it happens again.

3 Blood

HAEMORRHAGE

(for haemorrhage in neonates, see p. 182)

General

Internal bleeding is often more dangerous than external because it is less readily detected and controlled.

Diagnosis

1. The earliest sign of covert bleeding is a rising pulse rate. Older children may be restless and complain of thirst.
2. Continuing blood loss will lead to shock (p. 17), which in small children may ensue very rapidly.
3. Potential sites of serious internal loss are

   (i) peritoneal cavity
   (ii) retroperitoneal space
   (iii) pleural cavities
   (iv) gastro-intestinal tract
   (v) beneath capsules of liver or spleen
   (vi) around fractures (250 - 1000 ml for a fractured femur)
   (vii) into cranium (loss only likely to be serious in infant).

Management

1. If there is shock act urgently, as on p. 17.
2. If there is external bleeding stem it as follows:

   (i) apply prolonged pressure to wound (first check there is no glass in it)
   (ii) elevate the bleeding part (first check there is no fracture)

(iii) do not use a tourniquet (unless no alternative)
(iv) if there is arterial bleeding consult surgeon at once.

3. Assess total loss from

(i) history (acute bleeds tend to be overestimated, slow oozes underestimated)
(ii) signs of hypovolaemia (p. 18)
(iii) evidence of internal loss (e.g. abdominal distension; haemothorax on chest x-ray; haematemesis and melaena; swelling round fracture)
(iv) weight of blood-soaked clothes and dressings.

4. Express loss as proportion of total blood volume, which is c. 80 ml/kg. Figures for children of average size are:

age	*blood volume (ml)*
1 week	250
3 months	450
6 months	600
1 year	800
2 years	1000
5 years	1500
10 years	2400
16 years	4500

5. If *any* internal bleeding or if external loss >5% take blood for

(i) Hb (haemodilution takes several hours; an early sample serves as a base-line)
(ii) group and cross-match
(iii) platelets and clotting studies (if bleeding disorder possible).

6. If *any* internal bleeding or if external loss >15% (or >10% and continuing) put up a drip at once (veins may collapse later) and transfuse with matched blood. Replace *whole* of calculated loss not just part of it.

7. If child is restless or fearful, sedate generously.

8. Monitor pulse and blood pressure and inspect wounds regularly for recurrence of bleeding.

9. If thrombocytopenia, see p. 32.

Coagulation defects

1. A family history or a history of previous episodes is usual, but not invariable.

2. Coagulation defects typically cause
   (i) spontaneous bleeds into joints
   (ii) prolonged oozing (>24 hours) after open trauma, including tonsillectomy and tooth extraction
   (iii) disproportionate bruising after closed trauma
   (iv) spontaneous haematuria.

3. A haemophiliac requires urgent treatment if he has
   (i) severe bleeding from any source
   (ii) a fresh haemarthrosis
   (iii) *any* head injury (even if no evidence of bleeding)
   (iv) an extending haematoma in a dangerous site, e.g. neck or chest
   (v) a haematoma causing severe pain.

4. Transfuse as soon as possible with
   (i) cryoprecipitate (4 – 10 units depending on size of child and severity of bleed)
   (ii) fresh frozen plasma (if cryoprecipitate not available).

5. If child is a known haemophiliac, immediately contact centre that supervises him.

6. Keep in hospital until certain that bleeding has stopped (at least 48 hours for a head injury).

Epistaxis

1. Sit child up with head and arms resting on a table.

2. Sedate if at all agitated.

3. So far as possible clean nostril and check there is no foreign body.

4. Squeeze nostrils between thumb and forefinger for 5 min. Then wait for 10 min, and if still bleeding squeeze again for 5 min.

5. If bleeding continues try anterior packing:

   (i) soak some ½ in ribbon gauze in an equal mixture of 10% cocaine (as local anaesthetic) and $^{1}/_{100}$ adrenalin (as vasoconstrictor)
   (ii) insert into nasal cavity in layers, starting at the floor posteriorly and working upwards and forwards, packing gauze as tightly as comfortable
   (iii) remove after 25 min.

6. If bleeding still continues consult an ENT surgeon with a view to cautery or post-nasal packing.

7. Consider thrombocytopenia (p. 32).

Gastro-intestinal haemorrhage

See p. 53.

PURPURA

General

Purpura is taken here to include all haemorrhagic skin lesions from petechiae to ecchymoses. Some of its causes are very serious, and any child with a purpuric rash should be assessed at once in hospital.

Diagnosis

The causes come under three main headings: thrombocytopenic, vascular and mechanical. Associated clinical features may be helpful in diagnosis.

Thrombocytopenic purpura

Causes petechiae; often accompanied by epistaxis or bleeding from GI or GU tracts.

1. Idiopathic thrombocytopenic purpura — little systemic illness; sometimes follows minor infection.
2. Leukaemia — usually anaemia; often lymphadenopathy and hepatosplenomegaly.
3. Aplastic anaemia — anaemia.
4. Haemolytic uraemic syndrome — renal failure; anaemia.

(Also drug-induced thrombocytopenia, SLE.)

Vascular purpura

1. Henoch Schönlein syndrome — rash confined to legs and buttocks and sometimes extensor surface of arms; lesions initially erythematous and slightly raised; usually arthritis; often abdominal pain and haematuria.
2. Septicaemia, especially meningococcal — severe systemic illness; high fever.
3. Stevens-Johnson syndrome — widespread erythema multiforme; lesions of mouth and genitalia that may be haemorrhagic.

(Also scurvy, haemorrhagic measles and chicken pox, von Willebrand's disease.)

Mechanical purpura

1. Violent coughing, retching or gastric lavage — petechiae on face and neck.
2. Non-accidental injury — bruises of different ages and sometimes of characteristic shape (p. 118).
3. Coagulation defect — large bruises out of proportion to injury.

Management

1. Take blood for

Hb, differential w.b.c.	Culture
Platelets	Group and cross-match
Film	(if appropriate)

2. If transfusion required, use blood as fresh as possible.

3. If platelets $<25\,000/\text{mm}^3$ there is risk of intracranial haemorrhage, so

(i) give a platelet transfusion (if platelets not available use very fresh blood)
(ii) start steroids at once (unless cause is HUS).

4. If you are sure diagnosis is Henoch Schönlein syndrome, there is no specific treatment and hospital admission is only required if there is

(i) haematuria (risk of renal failure and hypertension)
(ii) severe abdominal pain (risk of intussusception).

5. Management of other causes

Septicaemia	Non-accidental injury (p.118)
Haemolytic uraemic syndrome (p.112).	Coagulation defect (p.30)

SEPTICAEMIA

(for septicaemia in neonates, see p. 114)

General

Septicaemia is more likely in a child who has predisposing factors such as:

Debilitation
Prolonged venous catherisation
Neutropenia
Nephrotic syndrome
Therapy with immunosuppressive or cytotoxic drugs, or with steroids
Previous splenectomy

But sometimes it can strike a healthy child out of the blue (especially meningococcal septicaemia).

Diagnosis

1. The typical features are

(i) rapid and unexplained deterioration in previous condition
(ii) high fever and tachycardia
(iii) initially peripheral vasodilatation, later vasoconstriction with cold, clammy, mottled extremities, proceeding to shock
(iv) rapidly developing rash (purpuric if organism is meningococcus)
(v) splenomegaly
(vi) acidotic respiration
(vii) paralytic ileus and vomiting.

2. The neutrophil count is usually high, but is unreliable because it varies.

3. If there is oozing from venepuncture sites, or other abnormal bleeding, suspect disseminated intravascular coagulation.

Management

1. If you see the characteristic rash of **meningococcal septicaemia** give i.m. benzyl penicillin before you do anything else; it progresses so quickly that any delay may be fatal.

2. If child is shocked, see p. 17.

3. Take blood for

Hb, differential w.b.c. and platelets	Electrolytes and urea
Culture (at least 2 ml into two separate bottles warmed before inoculation)	Clotting studies (if DIC possible).

4. Put up a drip for i.v. hydration and antibiotics. Give nil by mouth, and if there is an ileus or vomiting put down nasogastric tube and keep stomach empty.
5. Search for a source of infection, including chest x-ray.
6. Do a lumbar puncture if any suspicion of meningitis (always in an infant).
7. Try to identify the organism immediately by
    - (i) clinical features (purpuric rash suggests meningococcus; localised deep necrotic lesions suggest *Pseudomonas*; pustules suggest staphylococcus)
    - (ii) Gram stains from skin lesions, CSF or blood
    - (iii) review of any previous cultures.
8. Start antibiotics as follows (for dosages see p. 185):

Staphylococcus aureus	cloxacillin
meningoccus	benzyl penicillin + sulphadimidine
pneumococcus	benzyl penicillin
Salmonella	chloramphenicol
E. Coli	gentamicin
bacteroides	metronidazole
Pseudomonas	gentamicin + carbenicillin
unknown	gentamicin + benzyl penicillin
unknown in neutropenic child (often gut flora)	gentamicin + metronidazole

9. If meningitis is present as well as septicaemia give antibiotics as for former (p. 48).

10. If there is DIC consider heparinisation, in consultation with haematologist.

4 Central Nervous System

COMA

General

Coma may occur in the course of a serious illness when the child is already in hospital and the diagnosis known. This section deals mainly with the different situation where the child is brought in unconscious and the diagnosis is not yet established.

Diagnosis

Main Causes

1. Trauma
   - (i) head injury
   - (ii) fat embolism.
2. Poisoning
   - (i) alcohol
   - (ii) salicylate, etc.
3. Infection
   - (i) meningitis
   - (ii) encephalitis
   - (iii) cerebral malaria
   - (iv) septicaemia.
4. Seizures
   - (i) post-ictal state
   - (ii) effect of anticonvulsants (especially i.v. diazepam).

5. Metabolic disturbance

   (i) hyperglycaemia
   (ii) hypoglycaemia
   (iii) dehydration
   (iv) respiratory failure
   (v) renal failure
   (vi) liver failure (including Reye's syndrome).

6. Vascular disturbance

   (i) hypertension
   (ii) cerebral vein thrombosis
   (iii) intracranial haemorrhage.

7. Space-occupying lesions

   (i) tumour
   (ii) abscess
   (iii) haematoma.

Coma without preceding illness

Coma occurring without preceding illness is most likely to be due to:

Poisoning	Head injury
Post-ictal state	Intracranial haemorrhage

except in a diabetic when it is most likely to be due to:

Hypoglycaemia.

Management

1. Maintain a good airway

   (i) suck out vomit and secretions
   (ii) insert an airway or, if necessary, an endotracheal tube
   (iii) nurse child semi-prone
   (iv) keep equipment for intubation and inflation nearby.

2. If cause of coma uncertain check at once for hypoglycaemia (with Dextrostix) and treat it *urgently*, as on p. 72.

3. Check that respiration is adequate by noting rate, chest movements, air entry and colour; if in doubt do arterial blood gases and see *Respiratory Failure* (p. 11).

4. Begin regular observations from moment of admission, every 15 min at first, of

(i) level of consciousness
(ii) pupil size and reactivity
(iii) pulse and blood pressure
(iv) respiratory rate, depth and regularity.

5. Take blood for:

Hb, w.b.c. and platelets	Glucose Electrolytes and urea

(Drug assay, culture).

6. Put down nasogastric tube and empty stomach (keep sample for analysis if poisoning possible).

7. Test urine for glucose, ketones, salicylate (p. 84), and keep sample for later analysis.

8. If any possibility of head injury get a skull x-ray, and consult neurosurgeon *at once* if condition is deteriorating (p. 46).

9. If there is possibility of

(i) meningitis
(ii) encephalitis
(iii) subarachnoid haemorrhage

do a lumbar puncture, checking first that there is no evidence of raised intracranial pressure.

10. Consider i.v. mannitol or i.m. dexamethasone if you suspect cerebral oedema, which may accompany

(i) tumour or abscess
(ii) encephalitis

(iii) hypoxia
(iv) head injury
(v) cerebrovascular accident

11. Ensure scrupulous nursing care, with turning at least 2 hourly. If coma is likely to be prolonged or condition is deteriorating, arrange transfer to an intensive care unit.

CONVULSIONS

(for convulsions in neonates see p. 146)

This section deals with the management of (a) a child who is still convulsing and (b) a child who has just had a convulsion.

Child who is still convulsing

General

The two most urgent needs are:

1. To **prevent hypoxia** (which may cause permanent brain damage).
2. To **stop the fit**.

Management

1. Suck out vomit and secretions, and lie child on side.
2. Give 100% oxygen by mask, inserting an airway if necessary.
3. If any possibility of hypoglycaemia, correct it *urgently* as on p. 72.
4. Stop fit as follows:

(i) give i.v. diazepam in successive boluses of 0.2 mg/kg, pausing for 30 sec after each to gauge its effect (go cautiously after 2 boluses because of the danger of respiratory depression, especially if child has recently had phenobarbitone)

(ii) if you cannot get into a vein quickly, remove needle from syringe and inject diazepam 5 mg into rectum

(iii) if diazepam does not work give i.m. paraldehyde 0.1 mg/kg.

5. If convulsions continue intractably, call anaesthetist urgently with a view to paralysation.

6. Prevent child hurting himself

(i) do not leave unattended
(ii) remove or pad hard objects nearby
(iii) if he is biting his tongue, insert airway or padded spatula between teeth.

7. If further convulsions seem likely in the near future

(i) ensure immediate access to vein by putting up drip or inserting in-dwelling needle
(ii) start prophylactic anticonvulsant.

Child who has just had convulsion

Clinical

1. It is sometimes difficult to distinguish between a convulsion and other causes of transient unconsciousness, such as simple faints and cardiac dysrhythmias. A detailed history is essential.

2. Be alert for evidence of raised intracranial pressure:

(i) progressive history of headaches, vomiting, and ataxia
(ii) papilloedema and retinal haemorrhages.

3. Do not forget to take the blood pressure.

Diagnosis

1. If the child is febrile and is aged between 6 months and 5

years, the commonest cause is a febrile convulsion, but this may be clinically indistinguishable from a convulsion caused by meningitis (or encephalitis). Suspect meningitis especially if

(i) child is outside normal age limits for febrile convulsions
(ii) child seems seriously ill or has other features of meningitis (p. 46).
(iii) there is no discernible site of infection
(iv) convulsion is prolonged, asymmetrical or repeated.

2. If child is afebrile the commonest causes are idiopathic epilepsy or convulsions secondary to a brain lesion. Asymmetrical seizures are more likely to be the latter.

3. Temperature can be misleading:

(i) a child with idiopathic or secondary epilepsy may have a fit when febrile
(ii) a child who has had a febrile convulsion may have cooled down by the time you see him.

4. Other causes are as for coma (p. 37), with the addition of hypocalcaemia, hypomagnesaemia, rapid correction of hypernatraemia, and too rapid withdrawal of anticonvulsant therapy.

Management

1. Do a lumbar puncture if any possibility of

(i) meningitis
(ii) encephalitis
(iii) subarachnoid haemorrhage

but not if there is any evidence of raised intracranial pressure.

2. If the cause of fit unknown, take blood for estimation of

(i) glucose
(ii) electrolytes and urea
(iii) calcium.

3. If child is already on anticonvulsants, take blood for estimation of serum levels.

4. If diagnosis is febrile convulsion

(ii) give paracetamol 3 hourly till temperature back to normal
(ii) if temperature more than 38° C despite paracetamol, apply fan and tepid sponge
(iii) ensure good fluid intake.

5. If you decide not to do an LP initially, examine child again after 2 hours. If in doubt, do one.

6. If you suspect haematoma in a baby, do subdural taps (p. 173).

HEAD INJURY

General

Head injuries are very common in children. Two questions have to be answered:

1. Need the child be admitted to hospital?
2. Need he be referred to a neurosurgeon?

Admission to hospital

1. Admit the child for at least 24 hours' observation if

(i) injury was clearly severe
(ii) there was loss of consciousness or level of consciousness is declining
(iii) child has a bad headache or is vomiting repeatedly (some children vomit a few times after comparatively minor injury)

(iv) there are any neurological symptoms (e.g. ataxia, diplopia, blindness) or signs
(v) there is a fracture
(vi) there is a possibility of non-accidental injury (see p. 118)
(vii) child has a bleeding tendency (e.g. haemophilia, thrombocytopenia)
(viii) inadequate supervision is likely at home.

2. If child is not admitted the parents should be given instructions (preferably written)

(i) to bring him back at once if any of the above features develops
(ii) if he shortly goes to sleep to ensure that he is rousable 1 and 3 hours later.

Management

1. If comatose, see relevant items on p.38, *especially about respiration*.
2. Do not assume child's condition is entirely due to head injury, and always do a *complete* examination. Hypotension suggests an additional lesion or illness (though in infants may be caused by intracranial bleeding alone).
3. Be alert for injury to neck, especially if child fell head-first or was travelling in a car that crashed. When in doubt, immobilise neck until fracture has been excluded by x-ray.
4. Do a detailed neurological examination, including

(i) palpation of skull for a depressed fracture
(ii) measurement of head circumference (in infants)
(iii) examination of nose, ears and throat for blood and CSF (if there is rhinorrhoea check with Dextrostix to distinguish between mucosal exudate and CSF leak)
(iv) inspection of fundi (do not use a mydriatic).

5. Get skull x-ray as early as possible in case there is later

deterioration (ensure adequate supervision in x-ray department). *But base management on clinical assessment rather than x-ray results.*

6. Be particularly alert for extra-dural haematoma if there is

   (i) trauma in region of middle meningeal artery
   (ii) a lucid interval.

7. Record observations from admission, every 15 min at first, reducing to once hourly if no deterioration after 3 hours:

   (i) level of consciousness
   (ii) symmetry of limb movement
   (iii) pupil size, symmetry and reactivity
   (iv) pulse and blood pressure
   (v) respiratory rate, depth and regularity.

8. If child has a bleeding tendency

   (i) consult haematologist urgently
   (ii) if in doubt, give appropriate therapy (p. 30) as soon as possible even if there is no evidence of intracranial bleeding.

9. If child has a convulsion, stop it with i.v. diazepam and start i.m. phenobarbitone. Take into account effect of fit and of drugs when assessing subsequent level of consciousness.

10. Give antibacterial prophylaxis

   (i) for an open wound against tetanus (p. 52)
   (ii) for a compound fracture of the skull, which includes any fracture of the base, against meningitis (cotrimoxazole for 2 weeks).

11. If you suspect that there is marked cerebral oedema and there is little spontaneous improvement in 24 hours, give an infusion of mannitol.

Referral to a neurosurgeon

1. Refer as soon as possible any child with

(i) penetrating cranial injury
(ii) compound fracture of skull
(iii) depressed fracture.

2. Refer *urgently* if there is any evidence of an expanding haematoma, e.g.

(i) decline in level of consciousness (most important)
(ii) development of neurological signs, particularly asymmetry of pupils, ocular palsy and hemiparesis (carefully note sequence of signs, which may help locate haematoma)
(iii) slowing of pulse and increase in systolic blood pressure (late signs).

3. Never accept a diagnosis of brain stem injury without neurosurgical exploration, because similar signs can be produced by an expanding haematoma elsewhere that may be fatal if not treated at once.

4. Arrange meanwhile (if not yet done)

(i) skull x-rays
(ii) group and cross-match blood.

MENINGITIS

(for meningitis in neonates, see p. 144)

Clinical

1. In older children the features are as in adults, but in younger children they are less clearcut and may have been partly suppressed by antibiotics.

2. The usual features in a younger child are: fever, refusal of feeds, vomiting, drowsiness, irritability, dislike of being cuddled, even by parents (babies with other illnesses are comforted by

cuddling), increased fontanelle tension. There may also be a high-pitched cry, convulsions, head retraction and a 6th nerve palsy (late signs).

3. A preceding or concomitant respiratory infection is common.

4. Photophobia, neck stiffness and Kernig's sign are unreliable features in small children. Spinal stiffness can be detected in an older child by asking him to kiss his knees — normally achieved with ease.

5. Various rashes may accompany either bacterial or viral meningitis. A purpuric rash suggests meningococcal infection.

6. Meningism may be caused by tonsillitis, otitis or upper lobe pneumonia — but meningitis may accompany any of these.

Diagnosis

1. If you think there is a possibility of meningitis do a lumbar puncture and get CSF examined forthwith (see p. 162), except as in 3 and 4 below. If you are undecided, re-examine after an hour and if still undecided do LP without delaying further (complications are rare and the unpleasantness transient, but delay in diagnosis can be disastrous).

2. Before doing an LP always look in fundi for signs of raised intracranial pressure (this can be omitted in an infant whose fontanelle is patent and not tense).

3. If there is any suggestion of a space-occupying lesion, e.g.

- (i) progressive history of headaches, ataxia and vomiting over several days
- (ii) focal neurological signs
- (iii) papilloedema or retinal haemorrhages

there is risk of coning. Take further advice (preferably from a neurosurgeon) and, if proceeding with LP, remove only 1 ml of CSF.

4. If child is in a state of shock see p. 17, and resuscitate before you do LP, which may otherwise cause dangerous deterioration.

5. Take blood for

Hb, w.b.c and platelets
Culture
Electrolytes and urea
Glucose (to compare with CSF)

6. Do a chest x-ray if there is

(i) any possibility of tuberculous meningitis
(ii) meningism with normal CSF
(iii) a ventriculo-atrial shunt.

7. If initial CSF is normal but clinical features continue to suggest meningitis, consider a repeat LP after a few hours.

8. Always consider possibility of tuberculous meningitis.

Management of bacterial meningitis

1. Start i.v. antibiotics (give first dose i.m. if delay in getting up drip) as set out in Table 4.1.

2. Rapid identification of the organism may be available from Gram stain of CSF or by counter-current immunophoresis. Often

Table 4.1 Use of antibiotics for child with meningitis

Organism	*Antibiotics* (for doses see p. 185)
Haemophilus	chloramphenicol
pneumococcus	benzyl penicillin
meningococcus	benzyl penicillin + sulphadimidine
E. coli	gentamicin + ampicillin
Staph. aureus or albus	cloxacillin
unknown (child < 2 months old)	gentamicin + benzyl penicillin
unknown (child > 2 months old)	chloramphenicol + benzyl penicillin + sulphadimidine ('triple therapy')

Table 4.2 Common organisms of meningitis

Age	*Organism*
<1 month	various (see p. 144)
1-2 months	as for both adjacent groups
2 months – 4 years	*Haemophilus*
	meningococcus
	pneumococcus
>4 years	meningococcus
	pneumococcus

identification must await culture results, but if antibiotics have been given beforehand CSF may be sterile. The commonest organisms are outlined in Table 4.2. Children with ventricular shunts are particularly prone to infection by staphylococci (aureus or albus) or coliforms.

3. If the organism is not immediately identified, start antibiotics as for 'unknown', then

(i) modify when identification is made
(ii) continue a full course as for 'unknown' if no identification is forthcoming
(iii) consider stopping antibiotics if a relevant virus is identified.

4. There is usually no need for intrathecal or intraventricular treatment initially (though these may become necessary if there is poor response to i.v. therapy).

5. Give prophylactic phenobarbitone (oral or i.m.). If convulsions occur see p. 40.

6. In a baby, record initial head circumference to help in later diagnosis of subdural effusion or hydrocephalus.

7. If child has meningococcal infection ask GP to treat rest of household with sulphadimidine.

TETANUS

Clinical

1. Any wound can cause tetanus, but the risk is greatest from

(i) very dirty wounds
(ii) penetrating wounds
(iii) wounds with much tissue necrosis
(iv) wounds in which a foreign body is lodged.

2. The usual incubation period is 3 - 21 days, but it can be shorter or much longer. Sometimes there is no evidence of an infecting lesion.

3. Typical features are:

sometimes	stiff and painful muscles near site of infection
then	progressive muscle stiffness elsewhere, usually causing trismus and sometimes risus sardonicus, dysphagia, stiff neck and rigid abdomen
then	generalised painful spasms, provoked by stimuli, with opisthotonos and extended limbs (but flexed forearms).

4. The temperature is only slightly raised, but generalised spasms may make it higher.

Diagnosis

1. The whole picture is unmistakable, but parts of it might cause confusion with other conditions, e.g.

Trismus: cervical adenitis, mumps

Stiff neck: meningitis, drug-induced dystonia (e.g. phenothiazines, metaclopramide)
Dysphagia: rabies (either disease may follow a dog bite)
Rigid abdomen: peritonitis
Muscle spasm: tetany due to hypocalcaemia or alkalosis.

2. Probable severity can be estimated from interval between first symptom and onset of generalised spasms: if <36 hours illness will be severe.

Management

1. Give a large dose of i.m. benzyl penicillin immediately and continue parenteral penicillin for 5 days.
2. Give human antitetanus globulin 500 units i.m. as soon as possible (it only neutralises toxin that is not yet bound to neurones).
3. If there is a dirty, necrotic or penetrating wound arrange surgical exploration and debridement as soon as possible. Send swabs for Gram stain and anaerobic culture (often unsuccessful).
4. Put up a drip for sedation and hydration.
5. Sedate with i.v. diazepam, giving enough to prevent spasms, but not so much as to depress respiration.
6. If possible arrange urgent transfer to a unit experienced in treating tetanus. Travel at an early stage is likely to be less harmful than inexperienced management. If road journey would be arduous try and get a helicopter.
7. If there are respiratory difficulties or if illness is severe or likely to become so, arrange for curarisation and mechanical ventilation. If larangeal spasm supervenes, give 100% oxygen and arrange urgent tracheostomy.
8. Watch for urinary retention and catheterise if necessary.
9. Nurse with a calm routine in darkened quiet room.

Prevention

1. The organism is widespread, especially in soil. After *any*

wound give tetanus toxoid (0.5 ml i.m.) unless child has had full primary immunisation, plus a booster, within preceding 5 years (ensure completion of course if primary immunisation was deficient).

2. In addition, for a predisposing wound (as in *Clinical* 1. above)

(i) arrange urgent surgical debridement
(ii) give *Triplopen* i.m. × 1, followed by oral penicillin for 5 days
(iii) given human antitetanus globulin 250 units i.m. (into the opposite arm from the toxoid), unless child has had full primary immunisation plus a booster within preceding 10 years.

5 *Gastro-intestinal system*

GASTRO-INTESTINAL BLEEDING

General

1. Large gastro-intestinal bleeds are rare in children, and usually occur in those with a known predisposing condition. The management is the same as for adults.

2. Small bleeds occur fairly often, and while not serious in themselves may denote a potentially serious condition.

Diagnosis

1. Large haematemesis may arise from

   (i) peptic ulcer
   (ii) oesophageal varices
   (iii) bleeding disorder.

2. Small haematemesis may arise from

   (i) swallowed blood from epistaxis, severe pharyngitis, dental extraction, or cracked nipples (breast-fed baby)
   (ii) gastritis due to salicylate ingestion (even in normal dose), vomiting or stress
   (iii) oesophagitis, usually due to gastric reflux.

3. Melaena may arise from the above, plus

   (i) Meckel's diverticulum
   (ii) Henoch Schönlein syndrome
   (iii) small bowel polyps
   (iv) Crohn's disease.

4. Rectal bleeding may arise from

   (i) constipation or an anal fissure
   (ii) intussusception or volvulus
   (iii) polyp.

(Often, especially in babies, the cause is not found.)

5. Bloody diarrhoea may be caused by

   (i) entero-colitis (caused by various organisms, especially *Shigella, Salmonella* and *Campylobacter*)
   (ii) amoebiasis
   (iii) ulcerative colitis
   (iv) intussusception with incomplete obstruction.

(Also volvulus, pseudo-membranous colitis, and in neonates, necrotising enterocolitis.)

Management of large bleed

1. Take blood for

   Hb and platelets
   Group and cross-match
   Clotting studies

2. Put up a drip and, if blood loss profuse, a CVP line.
3. Monitor pulse and blood pressure half-hourly.
4. If diagnosis uncertain, consult surgeon and arrange endoscopy as soon as possible (barium studies are less informative).
5. If profuse bleeding from known oesophageal varices, infuse pitressin 5-25 units in 100 ml over 4 hours.
6. Unless surgery or endoscopy are imminent or child is vomiting, give plentiful fluids by mouth.

APPENDICITIS

General

1. Appendicitis is very common in children but may not present in the classical manner. It should be considered in any child with abdominal symptoms who still has his appendix.
2. The key question is not whether the child definitely has appendicitis, but whether the likelihood is great enough to call for laparotomy.
3. Appendicitis can occur even in the first year of life. The younger the child, the harder the diagnosis and the greater the mortality.
4. In a small child the main symptoms may be anorexia and vomiting, without obvious pain, and perforation and peritonitis occur early.

Differential diagnosis

Appendicitis – typical features

1. Pain is classically central moving to right iliac fossa, but can be elsewhere; it usually becomes constant and worse on movement, but it may be intermittent, mild or even absent.
2. Anorexia is usual and vomiting is common.
3. Diarrhoea or urinary symptoms may occur in pelvic appendicitis.
4. Fever is seldom >39° C (unless there is peritonitis), but often <37.2° C.
5. Persistent tenderness, usually in RIF but sometimes elsewhere, is the most reliable sign; in pelvic appendicitis tenderness may be most marked on rectal examination.
6. Guarding may be absent, especially in retrocaecal appendicitis.
7. Furring of the tongue is an unreliable sign, and the white blood cell count an unreliable investigation.

Table 5.1 Comparison of various conditions with appendicitis

Condition	*Typical features*	*Occurrence*	*Comparison with appendicitis*
Mesenteric adenitis	Preceding URTI	Very often	Quite often
	Pharyngitis and lymphadenopathy	Common	May co-exist
	Pain and tenderness	Fluctuates in position and time	Pain may fluctuate, but tenderness is constant
Urinary tract infection	Dysuria and frequency	Usual	Common
	Pyuria	Usual	Possible if pelvic appendicitis
	Loin tenderness	Common	Possible on right if paracolic appendicitis
Gastroenteritis	Pain	Colicky throughout	Sometimes colicky at first, but constant later
	Diarrhoea	Usually profuse	Moderate if pelvic appendicitis
Pneumonia	Flaring alae nasi and cough	Common	Unusual
	Grunting respiration	Common	Possible if peritonitis
	Chest signs	Usual	Unusual, but may co-exist

Table 5.1. cont. Comparison of various conditions with appendicitis

Condition	*Typical features*	*Occurrence*	*Comparison with appendicitis*
Meckel's diverticulitis	Bloody stool	Usual	Very unusual
	RIF tenderness	Common	Usual

Also consider infective hepatitis, Henoch Schönlein syndrome, sickle cell crisis, diabetic ketosis (p. 68), ovarian lesions, constipation, etc.

Other conditions

For typical features of other conditions, and their comparison with appendicitis, see Table 5.1.

Examination of abdomen in young children

1. Examine in mother's arms if possible.
2. Be unhurried and gentle. If he is asleep try palpating abdomen before he awakes.
3. Examine abdomen before ears and throat, which will start him crying.
4. Be sure your hand is warm, and if he does not like your bare hand try palpation through a sheet.
5. Start palpation away from RIF, and watch face for signs of pain.
6. If he will not relax give i.m. sedation and try again 40 min later.
7. A rectal examination is possible even in a small baby by gentle insertion of a well-lubricated little finger.

Management of possible appendicitis

1. Always do a complete physical examination (including a rectal).
2. Test urine as soon as possible for cells, protein and glucose.
3. An abdominal x-ray is not worth doing unless you suspect obstruction, but a chest x-ray may be needed to exclude pneumonia.
4. If appendicitis is at all likely consult a surgeon *without delay* because

   (i) delay in surgery can be dangerous in a child
   (ii) in doubtful cases he may want to observe over a period.

Whatever the initial decision on surgery get a consent form signed if the parents leave.

5. If peritonitis, see p. 59.
6. If dehydration or much delay before surgery, start i.v. fluids preoperatively.
7. If diagnosis is in doubt re-examine at least 2 hourly until appendicitis is excluded. Start hourly pulse chart and observations.
8. If at operation there seems increased risk of sepsis (e.g. perforation, purulent peritoneal fluid, local peritonitis), start metronidazole and cotrimoxazole (i.v. then oral) immediately after surgery.
9. If an appendix mass has formed, try conservative management (unless there is peritonitis):

   (i) give metronidazole and cotrimoxazole
   (ii) keep in hospital till mass clearly resolving
   (iii) if deterioration consider laparotomy
   (iv) arrange appendicectomy 10 weeks later.

PERITONITIS

Clinical

1. The features of peritonitis in older children are the same as in adults, the cardinal sign being a silent and rigid abdomen.
2. In very small children abdominal rigidity may not be detectable; usually there is grunting respiration and a worried expression.

Diagnosis

1. Much the commonest cause is appendicitis with perforation.
2. Primary peritonitis (pneumococcal or streptococcal) occasionally occurs in girls, especially with nephrotic syndrome.
3. Also consider tuberculous peritonitis, especially in immigrant children.

Management

1. If shock see p. 17.
2. Take blood for

Hb	Culture
Electrolytes and urea	Group and cross-match

3. Put up a drip and hydrate intravenously.
4. Put down a nasogastric tube; aspirate stomach contents then allow free drainage with hourly aspirations.
5. Consult a surgeon. Laparotomy is nearly always required, but rehydration may be necessary first.
6. Start i.v. antibiotics (cotrimoxazole and metronidazole if complication of appendicitis).
7. Give adequate analgesia (in consultation with anaesthetist if surgery imminent).

INTUSSUSCEPTION

Clinical

1. The usual age is 3–24 months (but can be any age).
2. Usual features are

   (i) intermittent bouts of extreme pain, with screaming, drawing up legs and pallor, but almost normal behaviour between bouts
   (ii) vomiting
   (iii) constipation then passage of bloody mucus (though if obstruction is incomplete stools may continue)
   (iv) collapse (later).

3. Typically a sausage-shaped mass is palpable in right upper quadrant, concave to umbilicus (but sometimes it may be palpable only *per rectum* or not palpable at all).

Diagnosis

1. Distinguish from

   (i) otitis media, causing bouts of screaming
   (ii) entero-colitis, causing bloody stools.

2. Do not be misled by fever and leucocytosis, which are usual in intussusception.

Management

1. If shock see p. 17.
2. Take blood for

   Hb — Group and cross-match
   Electrolytes and urea

3. Put up a drip and correct dehydration.

4. Put down nasogastric tube; aspirate stomach contents then allow free drainage with hourly aspirations.
5. Give strong analgesia (consult anaesthetist if surgery imminent).
6. Consult surgeon urgently.
7. Subject to surgeon's approval, consider a barium enema
   (i) to confirm diagnosis
   (ii) to attempt reduction of intussusception.

VOMITING

(for vomiting in neonates see p. 141)

General

Vomiting is a very common and non-specific symptom, especially in small children. This section deals only with vomiting of acute onset that is severe enough to require urgent attention or denotes a serious underlying condition.

Diagnosis

Table 5.2 outlines the various causes of vomiting — obstructive, cerebral and infective.

Management

1. Treat the cause of the vomiting.
2. Take blood for

   Hb and w.b.c.
   Electrolytes and urea

(Glucose, cultures, group and cross-match, poison assay.)

3. If shocked, see p. 17.

Table 5.2 Various causes of vomiting

Causes/conditions	*Typical features*
Obstructive causes	
Pyloric stenosis	Age 2–12 weeks, active baby, projectile vomiting after feeds, visible gastric peristalsis, palpable tumour, $Cl^-\downarrow$, $HCO^-_3\uparrow$
Hernia, volvulus, intussusception (p. 60), bands, adhesions, etc	Colicky pain, distended abdomen, bile-stained vomit, constipation, sometimes rectal bleeding (intussusception, volvulus), fluid levels on erect x-ray
Cerebral causes	
Meningitis (p. 46)	Fever, headache, stiff neck, bulging fontanelle in infants, CSF pleocytosis
Raised intracranial pressure (e.g. haematoma, tumour, hypertension, hydrocephalus)	Headache, effortless vomiting unrelated to feeds, papilloedema, bulging fontanelle in infants
Periodic syndrome	Previous episodes, no diarrhoea, sometimes fever, often abdominal pain, often acidosis
Infective causes	
Gastroenteritis (p. 63)	Fever, diarrhoea (sometimes not till later), colicky pain
Urinary tract infection	Fever, frequency and dysuria, often loin tenderness, cells and protein in urine
Appendicitis (p. 55)	Vomiting may be main symptom, especially in younger children
Peritonitis (p. 59)	Rigid, silent abdomen
Septicaemia (p.33)	Very ill child

Table 5.2 cont. Various causes of vomiting

Causes/conditions	*Typical features*
Metabolic causes	
Uraemia (p. 112)	History of renal disease or long-standing malaise
Diabetic ketosis (p. 68)	Polydipsia and polyuria, dehydration, acidotic breathing, pre-coma
Poisoning (p. 79)	

4. If dehydrated, see p. 74. In any case hydrate intravenously.
5. If appropriate try i.m. anti-emetics (e.g. prochlorperazine, metoclopramide).
6. If obstruction, ileus or precoma, put down nasogastric tube, empty stomach and allow free drainage with hourly aspirations.

GASTRO-ENTERITIS

General

Gastro-enteritis can usually be managed at home. Hospital admission may be required if

1. The child is dehydrated, or likely to become so.
2. Social circumstances make home management inappropriate.

Diagnosis

1. Always consider other possible causes of diarrhoea and/or vomiting, e.g. appendicitis, intussusception, urinary tract infection, Hirschprung's disease, ulcerative colitis.

2. Children with gastro-enteritis often have infection elsewhere. In particular consider possibility of meningitis, pneumonia, or septicaemia.

3. A child with gastro-enteritis may lose a lot of fluid into his gut before it begins to emerge *per rectum*. Often diarrhoea can be provoked by stimulation of the rectum with a thermometer or finger.

Management

1. Isolate and barrier nurse.
2. For assessment and management of dehydration, see p. 74.
3. Send stool for bacterial culture and electron microscopy for viruses.
4. Do not give antibiotics unless

   (i) there is additional bacterial infection that merits treatment
   (ii) the child is so ill that you suspect septicaemia (p. 33).
   (iii) the child has salmonellosis or shigellosis with severe systemic illness, in which case give i.v. chloramphenicol or cotrimoxazole respectively.

5. Do not give antispasmodics, which do not shorten the illness and may further weaken the child.

SWALLOWED FOREIGN BODY

General

1. Most of the foreign bodies that children swallow pass right through the gut without ill effect.
2. The possible hazards are

   (i) impaction, usually in oesophagus, leading to oedema and ulceration

(ii) if pointed, perforation
(iii) lead poisoning (rarely).

Management

1. X-ray to check nature and position of object (contrast studies may be needed if object not radio-opaque).
2. If stuck in oesophagus arrange removal urgently.

If in stomach or beyond – nonpointed object

1. No need for admission.
2. Instruct parents to

   (i) scrutinise stools and return if object has not emerged in 3 weeks
   (ii) return at once if abdominal pain, vomiting or melaena.

If in stomach or beyond – pointed object

1. Keep in hospital.
2. If in stomach arrange removal by endoscopy as soon as possible.
3. If endoscopy not available or if object beyond stomach, arrange surgical removal if

   (i) signs of perforation or obstruction
   (ii) no progress on repeat x-rays 5 days later.

4. If surgery required repeat x-ray *en route* to theatre.

INGUINAL HERNIA

General

1. Most inguinal herniae in children are reducible and asymptomatic and can be corrected surgically at leisure.

2. But the following need treating more urgently:

   (i) any inguinal hernia in a baby <1 month old (if it becomes strangulated, infarction may be rapid)
   (ii) a hernia causing intestinal obstruction
   (iii) a hernia that is not immediately reducible.

Management of a hernia not immediately reducible

1. Give nil by mouth; if there is evidence of obstruction, drip and suck.

2. If strangulation has occurred, arrange surgery as soon as possible.

3. If strangulation has not occurred try to reduce the hernia as follows:

   (i) sedate generously i.m.
   (ii) put legs up in gallows, or tilt bed head down
   (iii) get a consent form signed just in case
   (iv) wait 90 min
   (v) *gently* try to reduce manually.

4. If 3 works

   (i) check abdomen hourly for 6 hours for signs of infarction
   (ii) arrange surgery at next convenient time during this admission.

5. If 3 does not work, arrange surgery as soon as possible.

RECTAL PROLAPSE

General

Rectal prolapse looks alarming, but is not serious in itself — though it may indicate a serious underlying condition (cystic fibrosis).

Management

1. Reduce as follows:

   (i) wrap forefinger in soft toilet paper
   (ii) invaginate prolapse back into position
   (iii) extract finger leaving paper.

2. If this does not work, lie child prone with head down and try again an hour later.
3. If prolapse soon recurs, reduce it again and strap buttocks together with tape between stooling.
4. Prevent constipation.
5. Arrange a sweat test (if not done previously).

6 *Metabolism*

DIABETIC KETOSIS

General

1. Diabetes mellitus may present at any age, including infancy.
2. Severe hyperglycaemia may occur in

   (i) an undiagnosed diabetic
   (ii) a known diabetic out of control.

3. In children the onset of hyperglycaemia is often more rapid than in adults and is usually accompanied by ketosis.

4. A crisis is commonly precipitated by infection. The parents of a known diabetic may mistakenly stop his insulin because he is not eating.

Diagnosis

1. The features are usually classical: weight loss; polyuria and polydipsia; dehydration; drowsiness, followed by stupor, followed by coma; acidotic respiration; vomiting; sometimes abdominal pain and rigidity.

2. If no history is available there could be confusion with salicylate poisoning, which shares several of these features (see p. 84 for distinguishing tests).

3. When confronted with a known diabetic in coma always think first of hypoglycaemia (p. 72). Distinction should be obvious on clinical grounds but if not a Dextrostix will make it clear, and i.v. dextrose will do no harm.

Metabolic features

1. Dehydration may be as much as 15%. Rapid correction of this is more important than giving insulin.
2. There is often severe acidosis with pH sometimes <7.0.
3. Ketosis can be detected

    (i) by smelling acetone on the breath
    (ii) by testing urine with Ketostix
    (iii) by testing plasma with Ketostix (very useful when no urine available).

4. There is always a deficit of total potassium though serum K^+ may initially be normal. When treatment starts serum K^+ will fall rapidly (if not replaced) because of

    (i) dilution by fluid therapy
    (ii) re-entry of K^+ into cells caused by insulin
    (iii) re-entry of K^+ into cells caused by correction of acidosis.

5. Insulin is best given initially by i.v. infusion or, if infusion pump is not available or is unfamiliar, by frequent small i.m. injections. i.v. boluses and s.c. injections should not be used; the former give wide fluctuations in blood level and cause more rapid change in serum K^+, and the latter give unreliable absorption especially in a dehydrated patient.

Management

Immediate action

1. Put up a **drip** and run in 0.9% saline fast at c. 25 ml/kg/h (if shock start with plasma 20 ml/kg).
2. From other arm take **blood** for

    Hb and w.b.c.
    (polymorph leucocytosis is normal in ketosis)

    Electrolytes and urea
    Ketones (centrifuge and test plasma with

Glucose (and immediate Dextrostix)
Ketostix)
Culture

If child is very ill, also take arterial blood for gases and pH.

3. If child is vomiting or has depressed consciousness put down **nasogastric tube** and empty stomach.

4. Give soluble **insulin** by one of these methods:

either

(i) i.m. *in initial dose of 0.2 units/kg* regardless of degree of hyperglycaemia (if difficulty in drawing up very small volume dilute with saline)

or

(ii) by i.v. infusion (into the other arm) controlled by a pump at *rate of 0.1 units/kg/h* diluted in normal saline 1-2 ml per unit.

5. Unless child is known to have renal disease add $\mathbf{K^+}$ to main saline infusion at 20 mmol/l.

6. Search meticulously for **infection** (always get chest x-ray and examine urine) and treat vigorously with parenteral antibiotics.

Subsequent action

1. *Intravenous fluids*

(i) rate: 25 ml/kg/h for 2 hours; then 10 ml/kg/h until dehydration corrected; then daily needs (p. 181) and excess loss until full oral absorption is possible

(ii) type: 0.9% saline initially, changing to 4% dextrose/0.18% saline when blood glucose <11 mmol/l.

2. *Blood glucose*

(i) repeat estimation of blood glucose and electrolytes after 1 and 2 hours and thereafter as necessary (especially if deterioration in condition)

(ii) do a Dextrostix on each sample in case of an unexpectedly rapid fall in glucose
(iii) plot glucose results on a graph to predict roughly when level will be 11 mmol/l (change infusion to dextrose/-saline) and 8 mmol/l (stop i.m. or i.v. insulin).

3. *Insulin*

(i) repeat i.m. injections of soluble insulin *0.1 units/kg* every hour or continue i.v. infusion at *0.1 units/kg/h* until blood glucose comes down to 8 mmol/l and child is rehydrated
(ii) then start s.c. insulin on a *sliding scale*, 4 hourly at first, roughly as follows:

urine sugar	*units soluble insulin*
2%	wt in kg ÷ 3
1%	4
0.75%	5
0.5%	6

(iii) dosage required varies with individual needs and usually falls after the initial period.
(iv) all urine specimens *must* be double voided
(v) ketonuria persists 24 hours after cessation of ketone production because of tissue storage
(vi) be alert for Somogyi's effect (reactive hyperglycaemia following hypoglycaemia due to excess insulin).

4. *Potassium*

(i) modify amount given according to serum K^+, urine output and bicarbonate therapy
(ii) if serious abnormality of K^+ likely (or if child very ill) set up ECG monitor (hyperkalaemia — peaked T, then widening QRS; hypokalaemia — U wave, flat T, then inverted T, depressed ST).

5. *Acidosis*

   (i) this will correct itself in time (unless there is renal failure), and therapeutic correction carries complications (especially an abrupt fall in serum K^+), so do not give bicarbonate unless arterial pH <7.1
   (ii) for amount of bicarbonate, see formula on p. 77
   (iii) give slowly (over >3 hours).

6. *Urine*

   (i) record output carefully
   (ii) keep first specimen for tests (glucose, ketones, protein, microscopy, culture)
   (iii) if no urine passed: after 1 hour, stop K^+ (unless serum K^+ very low); after 2 hours, be wary about fluid overload; after 4 hours, consider renal failure (p. 112), and catheterise.

HYPOGLYCAEMIA

(for hypoglycaemia in neonates, see p. 148)

Diagnosis

1. The typical features of hypoglycaemia are

   (i) light-headedness, dizziness, anxiety, hunger
   (ii) restlessness, irritability, aggressiveness, or sometimes lethargy and drowsiness
   (iii) ataxia, clumsiness, slurred speech, squint
   (iv) tachycardia, sweating, dilated pupils
   (v) convulsions, coma.

2. The common causes are

   (i) insulin excess in a diabetic due to incorrect dosage,

eating less or later than usual or using more energy than usual

(ii) poisoning by alcohol, salicylate or paracetamol

(iii) ketotic hypoglycaemia (usually in thin boys aged $1\frac{1}{2}$ to 10 years, after a period of fasting)

(iv) acute liver diseases.

(Also consider insulinoma, glycogen storage disease, galactosaemia, etc).

Management

1. *Act urgently* if child is comatose or convulsing: there is risk of permanent brain damage.

2. If possible, first quickly take a blood sample for glucose estimation and do an immediate Dextrostix. (Be meticulous over the Dextrostix: use bottle opened <3 weeks beforehand; cover patch, or part of it, with *thick* blob of blood; leave it on *exactly 60 sec*; wash off blood with indirect and gentle flow of water; blot lightly; compare immediately with colour chart.)

3. If child is well enough, give him a sweet drink. If he is not, give 50% dextrose c. 1 ml/kg i.v. over 2 min. If you cannot get into a vein, give i.m. glucagon 0.5 - 1.0 mg.

4. If in doubt about diagnosis try a diagnostic test of i.v. dextrose. It cannot do any harm and may effect recovery.

5. If no improvement after 15 min, check blood glucose again and try more i.v. dextrose.

6. If child remains unable to drink adequately, put up a drip and infuse 4% dextrose/0.18% saline (at rate for daily need), or 10% dextrose if blood glucose continues low.

DEHYDRATION

General

1. The features of dehydration depend on

(i) amount of fluid lost
(ii) proportions of water and salt in that loss.

2. It is graded by the amount of fluid lost as a percentage of normal total body weight:

<5%	mild
5 - 10%	moderate
>10%	severe

3. Mild or moderate dehydration occurs in many conditions. Severe dehydration is usually found only in

(i) diabetes mellitus
(ii) pyloric stenosis
(iii) gastro-enteritis.

Clinical

1. Various points in the history may be a guide to the degree of dehydration, e.g.

(i) duration and severity of symptoms
(ii) fluid intake
(iii) urine output
(iv) last known weight.

2. Typical features are

(i) weight loss (allow for different scales and clothing)
(ii) dry mouth (but can be due to mouth breathing)
(iii) depressed fontanelle and sunken eyes

(iv) loss of skin elasticity (this may be hard to assess in a fat baby, whose skin cannot be lifted so readily; or in a thin baby, whose skin lifts easily even when well hydrated; or when the abdomen is distended; therefore judge by speed of relaxation of skin rather than ease of distortion, and do not only test skin over abdomen)
(v) tachycardia, low blood pressure, poor venous filling and eventually shock
(vi) tachypnoea indicating acidosis.

Hypernatraemic dehydration (serum $Na^+ > 150$ mmol/l)

1. Results from loss of water disproportionate to loss of sodium, from e.g.

(i) hypotonic diarrhoea
(ii) continued high solute feeds during diarrhoea
(iii) fever and tachypnoea with poor fluid intake.

2. High extracellular osmolality extracts intracellular fluid, so that circulating volume may be less impaired and elasticity of skin better preserved, though it may feel doughy or rubbery.

3. But cerebral disturbance is greater, resulting in lethargy, irritability and then convulsions. *Severe convulsions are likely if there is too rapid a change in osmolality during treatment*, so paradoxically the greater the degree of hyperosmolality the more slowly it should be corrected.

Management

Dehydration in diabetes mellitus

See p. 69.

Dehydration in pyloric stenosis

1. Because fluid loss is from stomach there is always alkalosis and hypochloraemia, and often hypokalaemia.

2. Take blood for

Hb
Electrolytes and urea
Group and save serum

3. Put down a nasogastric tube and empty stomach.
4. Put up a drip and infuse 0.9% saline for 6 hours then 4% dextrose/0.18% saline at rate to give daily need (p. 181) plus deficit over 24 hours.
5. Add potassium 20-30 mmol/l to infusion fluid as soon as serum K^+ known and urine passed.
6. Do not try to correct alkalosis; it will correct itself as rehydration proceeds.
7. Delay surgery until dehydration and electrolyte imbalance are corrected.

Dehydration in gastro-enteritis (and other conditions)

1. Take blood for

Hb and w.b.c.
Electrolytes and urea
Culture.

2. If there is shock, see p. 17.
3. Estimate

Fluid deficit
Daily need (p. 181)
Continuing loss (e.g. fever, diarrhoea).

4. If dehydration is only mild and child is retaining drinks, try oral fluids starting with a glucose/saline mixture (e.g. *Dioralyte*, or 4% dextrose/0.18% saline).
5. If child is not retaining drinks, or if dehydration is already moderate or severe, put up a drip and hydrate intravenously.
6. For intravenous regime, see Table 6.1.
7. Do not give potassium till serum K^+ is known and urine has

Table 6.1 Intravenous regime for rehydration in gastro-enteritis

	Type of fluid	*Amount and rate*
	Initially, before serum Na^+ known	
If shocked	plasma *then*	20-30 ml/kg fast
Otherwise	4% dextrose 0.18% saline	Daily need and *half* deficit over 24 hours
	When serum Na^+ known	
$Na^+ > 150$	4% dextrose 0.18% saline	Continue above rate for 48 hours
$Na^+ < 150$	4% dextrose 0.18% saline	Speed rate to give daily need and *whole* deficit over 24 hours
$Na^+ < 125$	0.9% saline for 4 hours *then* 4% dextrose 0.18% saline	Daily need and *whole* deficit over 24 hours

been passed. Then give at rate of 20-30 mmol/l according to serum K^+ and continuing loss (e.g. diarrhoea).

8. Acidosis will usually correct itself as rehydration proceeds so do not give bicarbonate unless there is

(i) renal failure
(ii) cardiac failure or shock
(iii) respiratory distress from overbreathing
(iv) pH <7.1.

The replacement formula is:

$$\frac{\text{base deficit} \times \text{wt in kg}}{3}$$

$$= \text{mmol } NaHCO_3 = \text{ml } 8.4\% \text{ solution}$$

This should be mixed in the infusion fluid and given slowly (over not less than 6 hours).

9. In severe dehydration repeat electrolytes and urea at 6 and 12 hours.

10. If convulsions occur during treatment

    (i) immediately re-check serum sodium and also check glucose and calcium
    (ii) consider meningitis and do a lumbar puncture if in doubt (dehydration may mask a bulging fontanelle)
    (iii) start phenobarbitone i.m.

In severe hypernatraemia (> 155 mmol/l) start phenobarbitone prophylactically as soon as Na^+ known.

7 Poisoning

GENERAL MEASURES

1. Suspect poisoning in any child with symptoms that cannot otherwise be explained, especially drowsiness, coma, over-breathing, tachycardia, flushing or unusual behaviour.
2. Ask parents to bring container and remaining contents, or sample of berries, fungi, etc.
3. Always assume child has taken maximum amount possible in the circumstances: parents' estimates are unreliable.
4. If uncertain whether substance is toxic, treat it as if it is.

Poisons Information Service

1. Do not hesitate to consult one of these centres:

Belfast	(0232) 30503
Cardiff	(0222) 33101
Edinburgh	(031) 229 2477
Leeds	(0532) 32799
London	(01) 407 7600
Manchester	(061) 740 2254
Newcastle	(0632) 25131 (drugs only).

2. These all maintain a 24-hour service and will advise on contents and toxicity of commercial products, on poisoning by drugs, berries, fungi, etc., and on management.

Management

1. If ingestion of toxic substance occurred less than 6 hours ago (longer for salicylate and iron), *empty stomach as soon as possible*, except

(i) for corrosives
(ii) for petroleum derivatives
(iii) when child is unconscious.

2. If child is unconscious

(i) see p. 38.
(ii) insert a cuffed endotracheal tube before gastric lavage.

3. If shock, see p. 17.
4. If respiratory depression, see p. 11.
5. For substance excreted by kidney (e.g. salicylate, phenobarbitone)

(i) maintain high fluid intake, by drip if necessary
(ii) consider dialysis (if available).

6. For slow-release tablets, give magnesium sulphate 300 mg/kg as a purgative.
7. Specific antidotes are available in only c. 2% of poisonings (see below), so further management is mainly supportive with particular attention to respiration.
8. Consider whether poisoning could have been deliberate (this is a recognised form of child abuse).

Emptying stomach

If possible use ipecac rather than gastric lavage. Ipecac induces vomiting in 95% of cases, empties the stomach more efficiently than lavage and is less traumatic for the child.

Method for ipecac

1. Give 15 ml of 7% ipecac syrup BPC (10 ml for child <18 months).
2. Wait 5 min.
3. Give 200 ml of water.
4. Wait 15 min.

5. If no vomiting yet, give another 15 ml of ipecac syrup.

6. If no vomiting after further 20 min and gastric emptying is essential, resort to gastric lavage.

Method for gastric lavage

1. Wrap child in sheet.

2. Select biggest tube that can safely be inserted, e.g.

For child <2 years	28 FG	17 EG
For child 2-4 years	30 FG	18 EG
For child >4 years	34 FG	20 EG

3. Mark on the tube the length that needs to be inserted; moisten it with water and insert gently but steadily as far as your mark.

4. If child vomits during insertion extract tube fully to allow free vomiting then resume (unless vomiting has been copious).

5. If child bites on tube keep jaws apart with an airway.

6. When tube is in position lay child on his left side with slight head-down tilt to bed.

7. Aspirate as much of stomach contents as possible with a large syringe; if no aspirate obtained make absolutely certain tube is in stomach.

8. Put in 50 ml of water and aspirate again.

9. Attach a funnel to the tube and pour in about 200 ml of tepid normal saline (1% bicarbonate for salicylate and iron); as soon as saline is in, lower funnel below child's head and allow fluid to syphon out.

10. Repeat till returning fluid is clear, which will usually take about 5 cycles.

11. Before extracting tube use it to introduce drugs if appropriate (e.g. desferrioxamine in iron poisoning).

12. Aspiration may occur even when child is conscious and can be more harmful than the ingestion; if child chokes or becomes cyanosed you should stop.

POISONING - CORROSIVES

(acids, alkalis, phenols, chlorates: e.g. strong bleaches, drain cleaners, etc)

Management

1. Do not empty stomach.
2. Allow no solids but give copious fluids, with neutralising substances if poisoning severe:

    For acid: 1% bicarbonate or milk
    For alkali: 2% citric acid or dilute vinegar
    For bleach: 2% sodium thiosulphate.

3. Look for burns in mouth (white or discoloured patches, becoming oedematous then ulcerated).
4. Give analgesia, topical (e.g. *Bonjela*) and parenteral.

If severe

5. Be prepared for

    Laryngeal obstruction
    Shock
    Perforation of the oesophagus

6. Hydrate intravenously.
7. Give parenteral ampicillin and cloxacillin.
8. Refer early to ENT or thoracic surgeon.
9. After recovery arrange follow-up in case oesophageal stricture develops.

POISONING - PETROLEUM DERIVATIVES

(e.g. paraffin, paint thinner, turps substitute)

General

The worst effect is pneumonitis, starting soon after ingestion because of inhalation or up to 24 hours later because of absorption.

Management

1. Do not empty the stomach.
2. Admit for observation for at least 24 hours.
3. Watch for evidence of pneumonitis (cough, tachypnoea, crepitations) and if in doubt do chest x-ray.
4. If pneumonitis seems likely give

    (i) steroids i.m. then oral
    (ii) ampicillin and flucloxacillin.

5. If severe, see *Respiratory Failure* (p. 11).

POISONING - SALICYLATE

Possibly dangerous dose >150 mg/kg

General

1. Salicylate poisoning is the commonest form of poisoning in children and also one of the most dangerous.
2. May result from overdosage of an already sick child as well as accidental ingestion.
3. Absorption and action are slow so that peak serum level may not occur for up to 6 hr, and maximum toxic effect later still.

4. In children under 4 years metabolic acidosis usually predominates; in older children there may first be respiratory alkalosis.

Diagnosis

If diagnosis is not evident from history it may be suggested by clinical features and confirmed by urine and blood tests.

Clinical features

Vomiting	Tinnitus	Restlessness
Diarrhoea	Vertigo	Hallucinations
Fever	Tingling of face	Convulsions
Sweating	Tachypnoea	Coma
Dehydration		

Urine tests

1. Phenestix goes brown-red.
2. Ferric chloride goes deep purple (boil first to eliminate ketones).

Blood tests

1. Immediate: test serum with Phenestix.
2. Laboratory: salicylate level.

Management

1. Distinguish from diabetic ketoacidosis (hyperglycaemia, ketosis, dehydration and coma may occur in either).
2. Empty stomach at once, even if ingestion occurred up to 12 hours beforehand.
3. Take blood for

Salicylate level   Electrolytes and urea

4. Clinical assessment is unreliable so make a rough estimate of severity by working out maximum possible dosage per kilo. Salicylate content of tablets is as follows:

Anadin 325 mg
Aspirin soluble paediatric 75 mg
Aspro Dover 300 mg
Aspro soluble 300 mg
Aspro Junior Dover 75 mg
Children's soluble aspirin (*Angiers*) 150 mg
Codeine 250 mg
Codis 500 mg
Disprin 300 mg
Junior Aspirin (*Angiers*) 81 mg
Phensic 380 mg
Safapryn 300 mg
Solprin 300 mg
Soluble aspirin 300 mg
Veganin 250 mg.

5. Plot on graph in Figure 7.1 the salicylate level against time since ingestion (mg/100 ml = mmol/l × 13.8).

If in asymptomatic range on graph

Press oral fluids.

If in mild/moderate range

1. Put up a drip and give 4% dextrose/0.18% saline at 30 ml/kg/h for 2 h, then 20 ml/kg/h, plus correction of previous dehydration.
2. Take arterial or arterialised capillary blood for P_{CO_2} and pH.
3. Unless already alkalotic add bicarbonate to drip to run in over not less than 1 h according to formula:

$$\frac{\text{wt in kg} \times (\text{base deficit} + 5)}{3}$$

$$= \text{meq NaHCO}_3 = \text{ml 8.4\% NaHCO}_3$$

4. Add potassium to drip according to serum K^+, allowing extra if giving bicarbonate.
5. Give vitamin K 10 mg i.m.

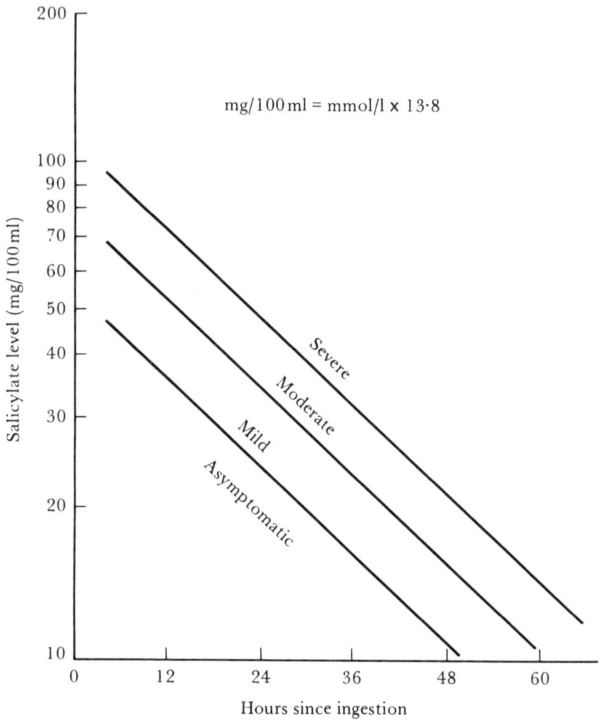

Fig 7.1 Salicylate poisoning (reproduced with kind permission of the author and publisher. From Done, A.K. 1960, Pediatrics, **26**, 800).

6. Check salicylate level, electrolytes, pH and P_{CO_2} at least 3 hourly.
7. Continue till plasma salicylate <40 mg/100 ml (c. 3 mmol/l).

If in moderate/severe range

As above, and consider haemodialysis.

POISONING - IRON

Possibly dangerous dose >40 mg/kg

Clinical

1. The early effects are usually

   Vomiting
   Gastro-intestinal bleeding
   Abdominal pain.

2. The later effects begin 6-24 h after ingestion and include

   Shock
   Acidosis
   Liver damage
   Convulsions and coma

3. There may be an asymptomatic period between early and late features.

Diagnosis

If iron ingestion is suspected, but not certain, it may be confirmed by

1. Positive ferricyanide (Prussian Blue) test on vomit.
2. Radio-opaque tablets on x-ray (but an x-ray may waste vital time).
3. Serum iron level (but do not delay treatment till you get the result).

Management

1. Induce vomiting (if not already copious) with ipecac.
2. Assess maximum possible amount of iron ingested. Iron content of tablets is as follows:

   ferrous sulphate 60 mg
   ferrous gluconate 35 mg
   ferrous fumarate 65 mg
   Folex 100 mg
   Fefol 150 mg

3. Unless amount ingested was trivial, observe child in hospital for at least 36 h.

If dose >40 mg/kg

1. Give desferrioxamine i.m. (0.5 - 1 g in 2.5 - 5 ml water).
2. In addition, wash out stomach using 1% sodium bicarbonate solution with added desferrioxamine (2 g/litre).
3. Leave further desferrioxamine in stomach (5 g in 100 ml) before withdrawing tube.
4. Take blood for

Serum iron (if >50 μg/100 ml expect serious effects)	Hb
Group and cross-match (if severe)	Electrolytes

If dose >60 mg/kg

As above, plus

1. Put up drip and infuse desferrioxamine at 15 mg/kg/h up to total i.v. dose of 80 mg/kg in first 24 h and 50 mg/kg in second 24 h (parenteral overdosage of desferrioxamine may cause shock mimicking the effect of iron poisoning).
2. If shock, see p.17
3. If severe GI bleed, transfuse with whole blood.
4. If severe acidosis, correct with bicarbonate (see formula on p. 17).
5. If evidence of GI damage, after recovery arrange follow-up because of possibility of stricture formation.

POISONING - TRICYCLICS

(e.g. *Tofranil, Tryptizol, Aventyl, Prothiaden*)

Possibly dangerous dose >10 mg/kg

General

1. The drug may have been prescribed either for an adult with depression or a child with enuresis.
2. The most serious effect is cardiac dysrhythmia.
3. Other effects are

Drowsiness	Agitation	Vomiting
Ataxia	Hallucinations	BP ↑ or ↓
Mydriasis	Convulsions	Coma.

Management

1. Induce vomiting with ipecac.
2. Set up ECG monitor.
3. Put up a drip (for giving drugs, diuresis is ineffective).
4. Tricyclics have an atropinic action which may cause extreme sinus tachycardia. If this exceeds 160/min (180/min if age <18 months) give

    (i) neostigmine 0.1 mg/kg i.m.
    (ii) pyridostigmine 1 mg/kg 4 hourly orally.

5. For other dysrhythmias, see p. 20.
6. Treat convulsions with i.v. diazepam.
7. If shock, see p. 17.
8. If cardiac arrest, see p. 24. Continue resuscitation for at least 2 hours because condition is reversible.

POISONING - PARAQUAT

(a constituent of certain weedkillers, notably *Weedol* and *Gramoxone*)

General

1. Extremely dangerous even in small doses.
2. Early effects are:

   Oral ulceration
   Vomiting
   Abdominal pain

3. Later effects are:

   Renal failure
   Liver failure
   Pneumonitis leading to pulmonary fibrosis.

Management

1. Immediately empty stomach with ipecac and then by gastric lavage.

2. Leave in stomach 200 - 300 ml 30% Fuller's Earth BP plus 100 ml 5% magnesium sulphate.

3. Test urine for paraquat (to 5 ml add a pinch of sodium bicarbonate and a pinch of sodium hydrosulphite; if it goes blue paraquat is present).

4. Put up a drip and start forced diuresis.

5. Telephone National Poisons Information Service (01-407 7600) for further advice.

POISONING - PARACETAMOL

Possibly dangerous dose >150 mg/kg

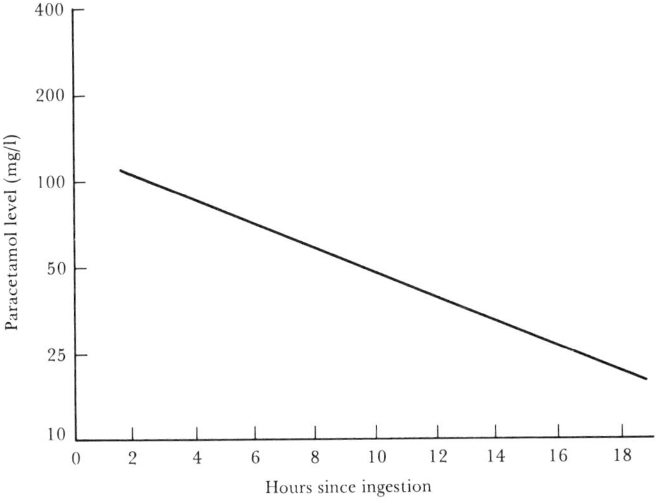

Fig 7.2 Paracetamol poisoning (reproduced with kind permission of the authors and publisher. From James, O. et al., 1975, Lancet, **ii**, 579).

General

1. Poisoning is unlikely from elixirs (e.g. *Calpol*) unless child drinks almost a full bottle (medium-sized bottle holds 140 ml = 3360 mg paracetamol), but adult tablets (e.g. *Panadol*) contain 500 mg each so that comparatively few can be toxic to a toddler.
2. The most serious effect is liver damage, which is dose-related and can be fatal. It does not become apparent for 2-5 days.
3. The usual early effect is nausea and vomiting.

Management

1. Empty stomach as soon as possible.
2. Take blood for paracetamol assay, base-line liver function tests and prothrombin time. Paracetamol level <4 h from

ingestion may be misleading, so repeat at c. 6 h.

3. If level is below line in Figure 7.2, serious liver damage is unlikely.

4. If level is above line, and ingestion was <15 h ago, give N-acetyl cysteine by i.v. infusion:

in first 15 min 150 mg/kg over next 4 hours 50 mg/kg over next 16 hours 100 mg/kg	diluted in 5% dextrose to give normal fluid needs.

(1 ml *Parvolex* contains 200 mg N-acetyl cysteine).

5. N-acetyl cysteine is most effective when given within 8 h of ingestion, but ineffective and possibly harmful if given >15 h after ingestion.

6. If poisoning is severe:

(i) check liver function tests and prothrombin time at 12-hourly intervals

(ii) if serious liver failure seems likely (e.g. if PT ratio > 2.5 on day 2-3) transfer to a specialist unit *before* it occurs.

POISONING - MISCELLANEOUS

Possible antidotes or special measures

See Table 7.1

Table 7.1 Various possible antidotes

Poison	*Treatment*
Alcohol	10% glucose infusion (to counter hypoglycaemia)
Amanita muscaria (fungus)	Atropine
Amphetamine	Acid diuresis
Atropa belladonna (Deadly Nightshade)	Neostigmine
Carbon monoxide	100% oxygen (hyperbaric if available)
Cyanide	Cobalt edetate
Digitalis	See p. 22
Distalgesic (contains dextropropoxyphene, an opiate analogue)	Naloxone
Lomotil (contains diphenoxylate, an opiate analogue)	Naloxone
Methyl alcohol	Ethyl alcohol
Opiates	Naloxone
Organophosphorus compounds (insecticides)	Pralidoxime + atropine
Phenobarbitone	Alkaline diuresis

8 Skeletal System

OSTEITIS

General

1. Infection is blood-borne and usually starts at the metaphysis of a long bone.
2. The usual organism is *Staphoccoccus aueus* (>90%), but several others are also possible (especially *Haemophilus*, *Strep. pyogenes*).
3. It is important to diagnose osteitis early and treat it vigorously because it can quickly cause serious damage to the bone.

Diagnosis

1. Onset is usually rapid (unless modified by antibiotics), and there is systemic illness with fever, anorexia and irritability.
2. An older child will complain of pain and tenderness, while a baby may

   (i) stop moving limb (pseudo-paresis)
   (ii) refuse to walk
   (iii) dislike being handled.

3. Initially there is extreme tenderness localised to one small area of bone. Later tenderness is more diffuse and there is overlying inflammation.
4. Inflammation of overlying soft tissue may resemble cellulitis, so apparent cellulitis over a bone in a child should always be regarded as osteitis.
5. Inflammation may provoke an effusion in the adjacent joint. Distinction from septic arthritis may then be difficult but is not vital since treatment is similar.

6. X-ray changes do not appear until at least 10 days after onset and usually consist of

(i) rarefaction
(ii) periosteal elevation.

7. Differential diagnosis is from

Trauma	Sickle-cell disease
Tumour (including leukaemia)	Scurvy
	Poliomyelitis.

Management

1. Take blood for

w.b.c. (nearly always polymorph leucocytosis)
ESR (usually raised; later changes are a guide to progress)
Culture (often positive)
Sickle test (negro children).

2. X-ray (may show other lesion, or provides a base-line if osteitis).

3. If osteitis probable on initial findings, start treatment with i.v. cloxacillin.

4. If diagnosis uncertain observe for 24 hours without treatment. If no deterioration in that time osteitis is unlikely. But if still in doubt start treatment.

5. Immobilise limb (back-slab of plaster of Paris is often helpful), and if possible elevate until inflammation has subsided.

6. Give strong analgesia because osteitis is usually very painful.

7. Consider surgical drainage (with culture of pus obtained) if

(i) intense pain not controlled by analgesia
(ii) clear evidence of subperiosteal abscess
(iii) no response to antibiotics in 48 hours.

8. Modify antibiotics in light of initial blood culture. If no growth and poor response to cloxacillin, add ampicillin.
9. Continue antibiotics for 6 weeks, of which 3 weeks should normally be parenteral.

ARTHRITIS

General

Some forms of arthritis in children require urgent diagnosis and treatment. Other forms do not, but, since they may initially resemble those that do, both categories are mentioned here.

Clinical

1. Usual causes of arthritis of acute onset are set out in Table 8.1.
2. Usual causes of hip pain of slower onset are set out in Table 8.2.
3. Hip pain is often referred to the knee.

Management

1. Any child with a painful joint and fever should be admitted to hospital until diagnosis is established, the most urgent need being to recognise pyogenic and tuberculous arthritis and treat them vigorously before they cause permanent damage.
2. Get x-rays of the joint, and possibly the chest. If the knee hurts, x-ray the hip as well.
3. Take blood for

w.b.c.
ESR
Culture

Table 8.1 Causes of arthritis

Condition	*Typical features*
Pyogenic infection	Usually in infants; often source of infection elsewhere in body; presentation similar to osteitis (p.94) systemic illness; purulent effusion; w.b.c. ↑, ESR ↑
Septicaemia (p. 33)	Severe systemic illness; often a rash; sometimes splenomegaly
Henoch Schönlein syndrome	Usually ankle or knee joints; little systemic illness; purpuric rash on legs; often abdominal pain
Haemophilia (p. 30)	Boys only; traumatic or spontaneous; usually previous bleeding or arthropathy; sometimes slight fever
Juvenile chronic arthritis	One or more joints; fever, often a rash; sometimes splenomegaly, nodules; ESR↑; rheumatoid factor positive 15% only
Rheumatic fever	Rare now in Britain; high fever; migratory arthritis; sometimes carditis, erythema marginatum, nodules; ESR↑, ASOT↑
Various viral infections (e.g. rubella, infective hepatitis)	Arthritis usually mild and self-limiting
Trauma	Effusion or haemarthrosis
Allergic reaction	Urticarial rash; often oedema; fever, but systemic illness not severe

Table 8.2 Causes of hip pain

Condition	*Typical age*	*Typical features*
Tuberculous arthritis	<5 years	More likely in immigrant children; systemic illness; fever; ESR↑; often infection elsewhere
Perthe's disease	5 - 10 years	No systemic illness
Slipped femoral epiphysis	10 - 15 years	Usually boys, especially obese; 20% bilateral
Benign hip syndrome (transient synovitis, irritable hip)	2 - 10 years	Usually boys; spontaneous recovery after rest

(ASOT, clotting studies, rheumatoid factor, viral titre).

4. Do a Mantoux.
5. If possibility of rheumatic fever do an ECG.
6. If there is an effusion consider aspiration (preferably under general anaesthetic) and send fluid for

Culture	AFB stain and culture
Gram stain	Cytology

Pyogenic arthritis

1. The commonest organism is *Staph. aureus* (others include *Haemophilus*, *Strep. pyogenes*, pneumococcus).
2. It is vital to identify organism, either from

   (i) aspiration of the joint (always do this if pyogenic arthritis seems likely)
   (ii) blood culture (take at least two).

3. If pus is aspirated

   (i) inject cloxacillin into joint
   (ii) consider open drainage if pus very thick.

4. If pyogenic arthritis seems likely start treatment at once with i.v. cloxacillin (as for osteitis, p. 95), modifying later when See. p. organism is identified.

5. X-rays are not usually helpful in initial diagnosis because specific changes may not occur for several days. But sometimes there may initially be widening of the joint space (by an effusion), and later narrowing of the joint space (due to destruction of cartilage), and rarefaction and then erosion of bone.

9 *Trauma*

SERIOUS ACCIDENTS

General

The order of priorities is the same as in adults:

1. Airway
2. Blood loss
3. Chest injury
4. Abdominal injury
5. Head injury
6. Skeletal injuries
7. Soft tissue injuries.

In children injuries are more likely to be multiple and deterioration is often more rapid.

Management

General

1. Get all clothes off immediately, cutting with scissors to minimise movement of parts that might be injured.
2. Do a quick initial examination of whole child (including his back) and a more thorough examination later.
3. Avoid movement of head or spine until reasonably certain there is no spinal injury.
4. Do not withhold analgesia: it will not mask a serious injury (though allow for effect on pupils and consciousness in head injury observations).

Airway

1. Remove broken teeth, dental plate or foreign bodies from mouth.

2. Suck out blood, vomit and secretions, and keep sucker nearby.

3. If child unconscious, insert an airway and if possible nurse on side with head down to reduce risk of aspiration.

4. If injury or subsequent swelling might cause respiratory obstruction, contact ENT surgeon urgently with a view to tracheostomy.

5. If any respiratory obstruction occurs give 100% oxygen.

Blood loss

See p. 28.

Chest injury

1. Look particularly for

   (i) flail chest
   (ii) pneumo- or haemo-thorax
   (iii) haemopericardium.

2. If any respiratory embarrassment give 100% oxygen.

3. If pneumo- or haemo-thorax compromising respiration, insert chest drain urgently (p. 166).

4. If flail chest, consult anaesthetist urgently with a view to mechanical ventilation.

5. If haemopericardium causing tamponade, aspirate without delay (try and get a cardiologist, but if not available do it yourself).

Abdominal injury

1. If any possibility of intra-abdominal injury consult a surgeon *early*.

2. Record girth measurements, at a marked place, every 30 min (but remember that acute dilatation of stomach may sometimes cause increase in girth).

3. Watch for signs of peritoneal irritation

   (i) tenderness and guarding
   (ii) absence of bowel sounds.

4. Be alert for splenic rupture if any blow to left side of abdomen or chest.

5. Unless injury and pain are slight, get either an erect (sitting) or lateral decubitus x-ray of abdomen to detect free gas from ruptured gut.

6. If doubt about bleeding into abdominal cavity, consider paracentesis.

7. Save first urine specimen and test for blood. If there is frank haematuria get an IVP as soon as possible

   (i) to see if there is extravasation of urine
   (ii) to check the other kidney in case nephrectomy is needed.

8. If injury to urethra suspected, try to pass a catheter into the bladder (normally easy in a child).

9. Re-examine abdomen at least hourly for the first 6 hours because bleeding may not manifest itself for some time.

10. Get consent for laparotomy if parents leave.

Head injury

See p. 43.

Skeletal injuries

1. X-ray all parts with external evidence of injury, including pelvis if any abdominal injury.

2. Splint unstable fractured limbs temporarily until proper reduction is possible.

3. Check for arterial occlusion, which requires urgent correction, especially

(i) axillary artery with dislocation of shoulder
(ii) brachial artery with fractures round elbow
(iii) popliteal artery with fractures round knee.

4. Allow for bleeding at fracture sites when estimating total blood loss.
5. If haemarthrosis, consult orthopaedic surgeon with a view to early aspiration.
6. If compound fracture, give prophylactic flucloxacillin.

Soft tissue injuries

1. Carry out appropriate tetanus prophylaxis (p. 51).
2. Test carefully for nerve lesions.
3. If injury clean and superficial, stitch it up yourself when you have a moment.
4. If deep, dirty, or involving nerves, tendons or vessels, arrange formal exploration and repair. Put on a temporary dressing meanwhile.
5. Always draw a diagram of injuries (you may have to give evidence about them a long time afterwards).

BURNS AND SCALDS

Clinical

1. Burns are assessed by their extent and their depth. In a child the 'rule of nines' cannot be applied because bodily proportions differ from adults; a skin percentage chart for children of various ages is shown in Figure 9.1.
2. Depth can be assessed as set out in Table 9.1.
3. Accurate assessment is often not possible initially.
4. Scalds, except when contact is prolonged or liquid is oily, do not usually cause more than deep partial thickness (DPT) injury.
5. Electric burns are usually full thickness (FT), at least in part.

Table 9.1 Assessment of depth of burn

Burn depth	*Skin characteristics*
Full thickness (FT)	Black or white Usually dry Insensitive Does not blanch on pressure
Deep partial thickness (DPT)	Pink or red Blistered or weeping Sensitive Blanches
Superficial partial thickness (SPT)	Pink Epithelium intact Sensitive Blanches

6. A burn or a scald may be a manifestation of child abuse, especially in a child under 3 years old.
7. The immediate problems following a bad burn are likely to be:

Pain
Hypovolaemia (from blistering, oozing and oedema)
Respiratory obstruction
Haemolysis
Infection.

Management

1. Give generous analgesia (morphine if burn more than trivial).
2. Draw chart of burnt areas and assess extent and depth.
3. Admit child to hospital if

   (i) extent >5% FT or DPT
   (ii) any FT or DPT burns to face, hands or feet, perineum or genitalia

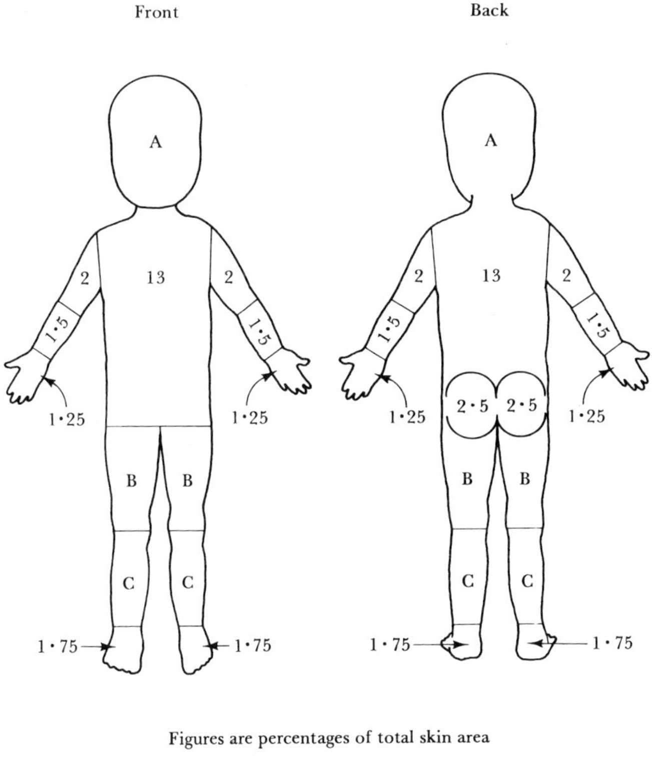

Fig 9.1 Skin percentages at different ages.

	Age (years)				
	<1	*1 – 5*	*5 – 10*	*10 – 15*	*>15*
A = ½ of head	9.5	8.5	6.5	5.5	3.5
B = ½ of thigh	2.75	2.25	4	4.5	4.75
C = ½ of leg	2.5	2.5	2.75	3	3.5

(iii) any possibility of child abuse
(iv) inadequate care likely at home.

4. If child is seriously burnt, if possible transfer to specialist unit at an early stage, *but i.v. infusion should always be started first.*
5. If shock, see p. 17.
6. If burn severe, take blood for

Hb	Group and cross-match.
Electrolytes and urea	

7. If burns involve face, or smoke was inhaled, be alert for respiratory obstruction and arrange immediate intubation or tracheostomy if necessary.
8. Weigh the child, if necessary in a nurse's arms.
9. If extent >10% FT or DPT put up drip and give

(i) **plasma**

($\frac{1}{2}$ *wt in kg* × *% extent of burn* = *X ml*
X ml every 4 h for 12 h from time of burn
then
X ml every 6 h for 12h
then
X ml every 12 h for 24 h

total = 7X in 48 h

plus

(ii) **0.9% saline** (for normal fluid requirements, see p. 181)

plus

(iii) **whole blood**
1% of blood volume for each 1% of FT burn

when >10% FT, give at once

when <10%, be guided by Hb.

10. Monitor blood pressure half hourly at first and chart urine output; if assessment of blood volume difficult consider CVP line and catheterisation.

11. If >10% FT or DPT allow nil by mouth and put down a nasogastric tube (ileus is usual).

12. Supervise toilet and dressing:

(i) clean burnt area (e.g. with warm cetrimide)
(ii) prick blisters and remove all dead skin
(iii) apply non-adherent dressing coated with bacteriostatic cream (e.g. *Flamazine*).

13. For burns in special sites

(i) involving eyes, consult ophthalmologist *early*
(ii) involving perineum, catheterise
(iii) causing tense oedema of a joint, consider skin slits to relieve tension.

14. If extensive FT burns be prepared for

(i) hyperkalaemia
(ii) haemoglobinuria; if present consider giving i.v. bicarbonate (sludging less likely at higher pH) and frusemide.

15. Give bacterial prophylaxis:

(i) penicillin i.m. 48 h then oral (against *Strep. pyogenes*)
(ii) antitetanus (p. 51).

NEAR DROWNING

General

1. After 5 min immersion in water the heart usually stops. After 10 min immersion recovery is unlikely.

2. The immediate effects of water taken into the lungs are:

   (i) asphyxia

   (ii) changes due to osmosis:

freshwater –	hypervolaemia haemolysis hyperkalaemia ventricular fibrillation
salt water –	pulmonary oedema hypovolaemia shock.

3. Later effects include

   (i) respiratory distress due to pulmonary oedema or pneumonitis
   (ii) hypotension
   (iii) dysrhythmias.

Management

1. Admit into hospital for at least 24 hours any child who has been immersed for more than a few moments, even if he seems to have recovered completely.

2. Check heart beat. If absent start cardiac massage (p. 25). Continue attempts at resuscitation for at least 30 min.

3. If breathing has stopped start artificial respiration *immediately* (seconds may be vital):

   (i) clear debris from mouth and pharynx
   (ii) tilt head down if possible, but do not waste time on postural drainage
   (iii) use mouth-to-mouth until equipment is to hand (p. 164)
   (iv) when possible intubate and inflate with 100% oxygen.

4. Empty stomach with nasogastric tube.

5. Take blood for

Hb
Electrolytes and urea.

6. If there is dyspnoea or cyanosis

(i) give 100% oxygen until P_{O_2} known
(ii) do arterial blood gases
(iii) if respiratory failure (p. 11) arrange assisted ventilation.

7. Unless not at all severe put up a drip for i.v. infusions and drugs.

8. If there is shock, see p. 17.

9. If there is pulmonary oedema give i.v. plasma (30 ml/kg) and frusemide.

10. Leave serum electrolytes to correct themselves except for

(i) gross hyperkalaemia:
give calcium gluconate 10% 1 ml/kg by slow i.v. injection
correct any acidosis (p. 77)
consider dextrose 25% 6 ml/kg i.v. plus insulin 0.5 unit/kg i.m.
(ii) severe acidosis (p. 77).

11. Monitor pulse and blood pressure half hourly for first 6 h. Set up cardiac monitor; for dysrhythmias, see p. 20.

12. Monitor urine output and check for haemoglobinuria (renal failure is unusual).

13. Give prophylaxis against

(i) pneumonitis with i.v. hydrocortisone
(ii) pneumonia with i.v. ampicillin and cloxacillin.

10 *Genito-urinary System*

HAEMATURIA

Diagnosis

1. The usual causes and their typical features are set out in Table 10.1.
2. A false impression of haematuria may be given by

   (i) a meatal ulcer in a boy
   (ii) vaginal bleeding in a girl
   (iii) the pigment from beetroot or sweets
   (iv) urate crystals staining the nappy.

Management

1. Admit child to hospital until more serious causes are excluded.
2. Monitor blood pressure.
3. Save all urine. Examine a fresh sample for casts, cells and bacilli, and send a specimen for culture.
4. Take blood for

Hb, w.b.c. and platelets	Creatinine
Film	ESR
Electrolytes and urea	

(Also consider protein, ASOT, C3 complement, clotting studies, group and cross-match.)

5. If there is renal failure, see p. 112.
6. Send throat swab for culture, and if there is tonsillitis give i.m. penicillin.
7. Arrange IVP (only urgent in case of trauma, see p. 102).
8. Cystoscopy is seldom helpful in a child with haematuria.

Table 10.1 Causes of haematuria

Condition	*Typical features*
Nephritis (commonest)	Often associated bacterial infection (especially streptococcal) or immune-complex disease (e.g. Henoch Schönlein syndrome, SLE); r.b.c. casts in urine
Urinary tract infection	Dysuria and frequency; fever; haematuria usually microscopic, but can be gross; also pyuria and bacteruria
Trauma	Trauma to loin or perineum; fractured pelvis; recent catheterisation
Foreign body in bladder or urethra	History not always admitted
Renal stone	Uncommon in children; ureteric colic; may be associated with cystinuria
Nephroblastoma	Age <5 years; palpable mass
Polycystic kidney	Family history; bilateral palpable mass
Clotting defect	See p. 30; r.b.c. casts
Thrombocytopenia	See p. 32; r.b.c. casts
Haemolytic uraemic syndrome	Preceding gastroenteritis; anaemia with schistocytes on film; FDP↑, platelets↓; r.b.c. casts
Renal vein thrombosis	Age >3 months; may follow asphyxia, dehydration or polycythaemia
Sickle cell disease	Negro children.

(Also tuberculosis, scurvy, sulphonamides, cyclophosphamide.)

ACUTE RENAL FAILURE

General

1. The diagnostic feature of acute renal failure is oliguria, which may be defined as a urine output of <300 ml/m^2/day (see p. 180: e.g. <125 ml/day in infant of 1 month;<200 ml/day in a 5-year-old).

2. Oliguria may be

   (i) pre-renal (usually due to hypovolaemia or hypotension)
   (ii) renal (due to renal parenchymal damage)
   (iii) post-renal (due to obstruction)

3. Renal oliguria in children is usually caused by

   Acute tubular necrosis (following hypovolaemia or hypotension)
   Nephritis
   Renal vein thrombosis (infant < 3 months)
   Haemolytic uraemic syndrome
   Acute on chronic renal disease (e.g. hydronephrosis plus plus infection)
   Toxins.

4. A pre-renal cause is suggested by

   (i) clinical evidence of hypovolaemia or hypotension and good response to their correction
   (ii) urine osmolality >300 mosm/l; urine Na^+ <20 mmol/l; urine/plasma urea ratio >5
   (iii) good response to frusemide 4 mg/kg i.v. (avoid mannitol if possible).

5. A post-renal cause may be revealed by

   Palpation of a full bladder (but avoid this unless essential)
   Catheterisation
   High dose IVP.

Management

1. The principles are

   (i) exclude pre-renal and post-renal causes
   (ii) identify renal cause and treat it if possible
   (iii) maintain electrolyte balance until kidneys resume adequate function.

2. Take blood for

Hb, w.b.c., platelets	Creatinine
Film	Calcium and phosphate
Electrolytes and urea	Culture

(Also protein, ASOT, C3 complement, FDP, ESR, group, cross-match).

3. Save all urine and do these tests:

Microscopy	Osmolality
Protein	Culture
Electrolytes and urea	

4. Avoid catheterisation when possible, but do it temporarily if

   (i) uncertain whether there is a full bladder
   (ii) no urine specimen available after 6 h
   (iii) dialysis required.

5. Record exact weight of child and keep very accurate fluid chart. If in serious doubt about circulating fluid volume consider CVP line.

6. Allow fluid intake equivalent to

   (i) insensible loss (c. 1 ml/kg/h; more if febrile or overbreathing)
   (ii) urine output in previous 24 h
   (iii) fluid content of vomit and stools.

7. Food and drink:

   (i) give fluids orally unless child vomiting or unable to drink
   (ii) use high calorie fluids (e.g. oral *Caloreen* or i.v. 10% dextrose) to minimise tissue breakdown
   (iii) restrict protein to <1 g/kg/day
   (iv) avoid cow's milk, which has a high concentration of solute
   (v) avoid drinks and sweets that contain a lot of potassium (e.g. fruit juice, chocolate).

8. If there is hyperkalaemia consider oral or rectal calcium polystyrene sulphonate resin (*Resonium* A) 0.5 g/kg, repeated 12 hourly.

9. If there is severe acidosis consider oral or i.v. bicarbonate (p. 77), but avoid overload of sodium.

10. Consider peritoneal dialysis (which is usually easier and more effective in a child than in an adult) if

   (i) serum K^+ >7 mmol/l despite attempts at reduction
   (ii) urea >65 mmol/l or rising >16 mmol/l per 24 h
   (iii) bicarbonate <13 mmol/l, uncorrectable because of Na^+ overload
   (iv) hypertension or fluid retention
   (v) clinical deterioration, especially in CNS (e.g. drowsiness, convulsions).

11. Treat any infection vigorously, especially of urinary tract (using reduced dose if drugs excreted by kidney).

PAINFUL TESTIS

Clinical

1. *A painful testis should always be regarded as a surgical emergency until proved otherwise.*

2. The usual causes are:

Torsion of the cord	Haematoma
Torsion of a testicular appendage	Epididymo-orchitis.

3. If torsion of cord is left uncorrected for more than a few hours it results in the loss of the testis. It may occur

(i) at any age, even in the neonate
(ii) in an undescended testis
(iii) following trauma (and be confused with a haematoma).

4. Epididymo-orchitis is uncommon in childhood. Fever and dysuria are not diagnostic of it, for they may also accompany torsion of cord.

Management

1. Always admit child to hospital.
2. Unless another diagnosis is certain (e.g. mumps orchitis or obvious haematoma) assume diagnosis is torsion of cord and consult surgeon *immediately*.
3. *Never* give a trial of antibiotics.
4. In doubtful cases surgery is the safest policy: the risk of exploring an infected organ is far less than that of treating infarction with antibiotics.

PARAPHIMOSIS

General

1. Paraphimosis can occur at any age. It is particularly likely to follow attempts to retract a tight foreskin.
2. It should always be corrected as soon as possible because the longer it is left the more difficult correction becomes.

Management

1. Give strong analgesia (e.g. morphine) i.m.
2. Grasp end of penis steadily for 2 min to squeeze back as much oedema as possible.
3. Try to slide foreskin forwards over glans.
4. If this does not work, arrange for dorsal slit and reduction to be done under general anaesthesia as soon as possible.
5. Arrange for circumcision at a later date.

11 *Parents*

THE WORRIED PARENT

General

1. Mothers sometimes bring a baby to an Accident Department because they are worried about non-specific symptoms such as crying, lethargy or poor feeding. It is important to recognise those babies who have a serious illness, and to be able to reassure the parents of the majority who have not.

2. The mother is usually the best judge of the health of her baby, especially if she is sensible and experienced. If she says he is ill she is probably right.

Clinical

1. If a baby is screaming look particularly for

Otitis media (p. 13)
Meningitis (p. 46)
Intestinal obstruction, especially from intussusception or inguinal hernia
Maternal anxiety, which can be a cause as well as a result of a baby's screaming.

2. If a baby is lethargic and off his feeds look particularly for

Meningitis (p.46)
Pneumonia (p. 6)
Septicaemia (p. 33)
Urinary tract infection
Early gastro-enteritis.

3. Worrying features include

Drowsiness and lack of interest in surroundings
An unusual cry, and reluctance to be comforted by cuddling
A very high temperature (or hypothermia)
A rash, especially if purpuric (p. 31)
A tense fontanelle (when not crying)
Poor peripheral circulation, and tachycardia when quiet
Tachypnoea

Management

1. If there is any possibility of a serious condition admit the baby to the ward, preferably with his mother.
2. Be more ready to admit the baby if

(i) home circumstances are poor
(ii) another child in the family has had a serious illness or has died unexpectedly (e.g. cot death)
(iii) the mother seems near the end of her tether.

3. If the problem seems to arise from maternal anxiety

(i) take time listening to the mother's worries
(ii) get in touch with family doctor, health visitor and social worker (if involved)
(iii) if necessary admit baby to the ward to give mother a break.

CHILD ABUSE

General

1. Child abuse is relatively common, affecting at least 1 child

per 1000. The usual age is under 3 years, but may be older. It may occur in any social class and be inflicted by either parent or by another care-taker.

2. Child abuse should be borne in mind in any child under 3 who has an injury other than from a traffic accident. It may also take the form of a burn or a scald or an overdose.

3. It is vital to recognise it because

(i) the recurrence rate is high
(ii) siblings may also be at risk
(iii) it is a very serious condition, with c. 10% mortality and c. 30% brain damage.

Clinical

1. The typical history may include

(i) explanation varying or inconsistent with injury
(ii) delay in seeking medical attention
(iii) previous incidents involving this child or a sibling
(iv) parents who had a disturbed childhood themselves, are immature, emotionally disordered or socially isolated
(v) a baby who was unwanted or required special care as a neonate.

2. The typical signs include

(i) injuries of different ages
(ii) finger marks, especially on head, trunk and arms (from grasping and shaking)
(iii) black eyes or purple ears
(iv) torn lingual frenulum (from forcing bottle into mouth)
(v) oval bruises with a clear centre (bite marks)
(vi) cigarette burns, or burns on buttocks and perineum (from placing on hot object)
(vii) retinal haemorrhages
(viii) evidence of poor care.

3. Subdural haematomata are commonly present and are usually bilateral. They are usually caused by violent shaking so not necessarily associated with a fracture. Typical symptoms are irritability, vomiting, convulsions or unexplained malaise; there may often be retinal haemorrhages and sometimes a bulging fontanelle.

4. Typical x-ray signs include

(i) multiple bony lesions, characteristically of different ages
(ii) epiphyseal displacement or metaphyseal fragmentation
(iii) avulsion of part of provisional zone of calcification
(iv) a double contour line of periosteum (not evident till 2 weeks after injury) followed by cortical thickening
(v) a spiral fracture in a small child.

Management of suspected child abuse

1. Admit child to hospital if possible.
2. Discuss with consultant paediatrician at once: he may want to do all interviewing himself.
3. Record in detail initial explanation given by parents and take a very full social history.
4. Draw diagram of any injuries, with descriptive notes, including estimate of their age.
5. Get photograph as soon as possible (bruises soon fade).
6. Get skeletal survey (remember it may need repeating in 2 weeks' time).
7. If there is bruising take blood for

Hb and platelets.
Clotting tests.

8. Find out if there has been any previous suspicion of child abuse in family by telephoning

(i) family doctor
(ii) health visitor

(iii) Social Services Department, who keep a register of abused children.

9. Ask nursing staff to observe child's behaviour on the ward, and to keep record of parental visits and inquiries.

10. If parents insist on taking child home in circumstances which you consider dangerous, contact Social Services Department at once and ask them to obtain a 'Place of Safety Order', which makes it illegal to remove child from hospital.

12 *Neonatal Emergencies*

BIRTH ASPHYXIA

General

1. Birth asphyxia may be defined as hypoxia of a baby at birth, resulting from inadequate oxygenation before, during or after delivery.

2. Ante- or intra-partum asphyxia predisposes to post-partum asphyxia by depressing the respiratory centre.

3. A newborn baby can tolerate hypoxia better than an adult, and normal survival is possible even after a long period (e.g. 20 min) of asphyxia. But resuscitation should be started as early as possible to reduce the risk of brain damage.

4. Asphyxia is more likely following:

Caesarian section
Difficult instrumental delivery
Malpresentation
Ante-partum haemorrhage obstruction of the cord
Heavy sedation of the mother

Clinical

1. Ante-partum asphyxia may be detected by signs of fetal distress:

(i) slowing of the heart rate
(ii) meconium staining of the liquor.

2. At birth a severely asphyxiated baby

(i) looks pale with deeply cyanosed lips and tongue
(ii) lies flaccid and motionless

(iii) makes no regular respiratory effort — though it may gasp intermittently
(iv) has a low (<80) or falling heart rate — this is the best indication of the duration of asphyxia
(v) becomes increasingly acidotic — which depresses the heart.

Management

Advance measures

1. Make yourself thoroughly familiar with the lay-out of the delivery room and with the resuscitation equipment.
2. Make regular checks of the equipment. It should include:

Resuscitation trolley (with heater, clock and IPPV apparatus)
Mucus extractor
Laryngoscope (preferably two)
Endotracheal tubes (2.5, 3.0 and 3.5 mm)
Fine catheter (to pass down ET tube)
Connector (to link ET tube with IPPV)
Bag and mask
Infant airway
Umbilical catheter
Scalpel blade
Silk stitch (with needle)
Ampoules of 8.4% bicarbonate (c. 5 ml), 20 %dextrose (c. 10 ml) and naloxone (paediatric and adult strength)
Syringes and needles

3. Ask obstetricians and midwives always to give you as much warning as possible when they are expecting a difficult delivery or an asphyxiated baby.
4. When called to a delivery check

Equipment is all present
Laryngoscope light works
Oxygen is connected
Trolley heater is on
Warm cot or incubator at hand

Pressure relief valve ('blow off') is working	Drugs mother has had in the last few hours

When baby is born

1. Start the clock.
2. Quickly wrap baby with a warm towel and place him on another towel under the heater.
3. Suck out mouth, nose and pharynx with mucus extractor.
4. Count heart rate with a stethoscope.
5. Keep him as warm as possible throughout.

Intubation

(For technique see p. 168.)

1. Intubate baby if

   (i) heart beat at birth is absent or <40 and not picking up
   (ii) heart rate at one minute is <100 and not picking up
   (iii) there is no respiratory effort at one minute
   (iv) regular respiration is not established at 2 min
   (v) there is a risk of aspiration of meconium.

2. Before inflating lungs suck out trachea by means of catheter passed down ET tube. Do this very thoroughly if meconium is present (if meconium is thick suck it directly up ET tube, then re-intubate).
3. If you have tried and failed to intubate for more than 60 sec, ventilate with oxygen by bag and mask for a short while then try again (or give mouth-to-mouth ventilation, see p. 164).
4. When ET tube is in position and trachea sucked out, start IPPV at c. 40 inflations/min.
5. Check that chest movements and air entry are symmetrical. If only right side of chest moves, tube is probably in right main bronchus — try withdrawing it 1 cm.
6. After 30 sec of IPPV pause to see if spontaneous respiration is

established and adequate; if it is, stop IPPV but leave ET tube *in situ* for another minute.

7. If respiration is inadequate after 5 min and mother was given opiates within 4 hours of delivery, give **naloxone**:

either

(i) 0.1 - 0.2 mg (0.25 - 0.5 ml adult *Narcan*) i.m. (massage to encourage absorption)

or

(ii) 0.02 - 0.04 mg (1 - 2 ml paediatric *Narcan*) i.v. by umbilical catheter (see p. 177 for technique) flushed in with 20% dextrose.

Cardiac massage

(For technique, see p, 25.)

1. If heart beat is absent or <30 at any time begin cardiac massage at once.

2. If you are alone, massage for 10 beats, then intubate and start inflating lungs, then continue both together. If possible get someone else to do the cardiac massage for you (make sure they are doing it correctly).

3. If heart beat still absent or <30 after 2 min of massage, inject 8.4% bicarbonate 2-4 ml by cardiac puncture (insert needle through c. 5th intercostal space just to left of sternum; ensure position in ventricle by ready back-flow of blood).

4. Survival without severe brain damage is unlikely if

(i) an adequate heart beat is not established after 20 mins of cardiac massage

(ii) *regular* respiration (not gasps) is not established after 30 min of adequate heart beat (after eliminating possible effects of maternal drugs).

CONGENITAL ABNORMALITIES REQUIRING URGENT ACTION

Oesophageal atresia

(Incidence c. 1/3000)

1. Suspect if

   (i) there is polyhydramnios
   (ii) baby drools excessively
   (iii) baby frequently splutters and goes blue.

2. Diagnose by trying to pass catheter of mucus extractor into stomach (a finer catheter may curl up) and testing with litmus fluid obtained.

Management

1. Do not feed.
2. Aspirate saliva every 15 min.
3. Nurse in a sitting position (to prevent reflux of gastric fluid).
4. Check for associated anomalies (especially imperforate anus).
5. Send to neonatal surgical unit as soon as possible (still sitting).

Diaphragmatic hernia

(Incidence c. 1/2200)

1. Suspect if

   (i) baby fails to breath adequately or has immediate respiratory distress
   (ii) lungs do not inflate properly with IPPV
   (iii) apex beat is displaced to right (herniation is on left in 90%).

2. Diagnose by chest x-ray (remember bowel may contain no gas at first).

Management

1. Keep intubated, and use IPPV by hand or machine at higher than usual pressure if necessary.
2. Do not inflate with a mask (forces air into stomach).
3. Put down nasogastric tube, leave drainage open and aspirate stomach every 10 min.
4. Nurse on side with good lung uppermost and feet tilted down.
5. Send to neonatal surgical unit as soon as possible (with a doctor in attendance).

Exomphalos

(Incidence c. 1/5000)

1. If lesion is dirty clean gently with warm sterile saline.
2. Cover it with sterile polythene or moist saline packs kept in place with strapping.
3. Put down nasogastric tube, leave drainage open and aspirate stomach every 10 min.
4. Check for associated anomalies.
5. If sac has ruptured start parenteral gentamicin and benzyl penicillin.
6. Send to neonatal surgical unit as soon as possible.

Myelomeningocele

(Incidence c. 1/400.)

1. If lesion is dirty, clean gently with warm sterile saline. Cover it with sterile polythene or moist saline packs kept in place with strapping.
2. Make a careful assessment of the features that determine the decision on surgical treatment:

(i) site and extent of lesion
(ii) its covering. (Skin? Meninges? Nil?)
(iii) integrity of nerve supply below it (assess by deformity of legs; spontaneous movement of each muscle group; tone and reflexes; response to pain; anal tone and reflex)
(iv) associated anomalies, especially hydrocephalus (measure head circumference) and kyphoscoliosis.

3. Consult neuro- or neonatal surgeon urgently.
4. If it is decided to treat surgically and lesion is open or oozing CSF, start parenteral gentamicin and benzyl penicillin.

Pierre Robin syndrome

(Incidence c. 1/1500.)

1. Suspect if there is

(i) small lower jaw
(ii) respiratory obstruction immediately after birth.

2. Respiratory obstruction is caused by tongue slipping back into pharynx and can be relieved by

(i) placing baby prone

or

(ii) inserting an airway

or

(iii) intubation (may be difficult - introducer may be necessary).

3. Look for associated cleft palate and microcephaly.
4. Surgery is not normally required in neonatal period, but baby may have to be nursed prone for some time.

Cyanotic heart disease

(Incidence c. 1/1000)

1. Heart lesions that cause cyanosis in the neonatal period are usually soon fatal if uncorrected. Prompt recognition and early surgical intervention may be life-saving.

2. The cyanosis of heart disease must be distinguished from

 (i) the cyanosis of respiratory disease
 (ii) peripheral cyanosis (very common for the first 12 hours after birth)
 (iii) 'traumatic cyanosis' (an impression of cyanosis given by congestion and petechiae resulting from a difficult delivery).

3. There may not be a murmur.

Management

1. If diagnosis in doubt, get chest x-ray, ECG, blood gases (p. 153).
2. Give 100% oxygen.
3. Send immediately to paediatric cardiological unit.

SMALL BABIES

General

1. Low birth weight is by definition <2.5 kg. It may arise from

 (i) prematurity (pre-term)
 (ii) intra-uterine malnutrition (light-for-dates)
 (iii) a combination of both.

2. It is important to distinguish these because they bring different problems.
3. A baby is regarded as preterm if gestation is <37 weeks.
4. A baby is regarded as light-for-dates if birth weight is below

the 10th centile for gestation. This is an arbitrary definition because

(i) not all such babies have suffered intra-uterine malnutrition: they may also be small because of heredity, congenital infection or abnormality
(ii) some babies *above* this weight may have suffered from intra-uterine malnutrition: they look long, thin and scraggy.

Management

1. Keep baby warm.
2. Assess gestation by method given on p. 175, which is simple reasonably accurate and causes little disturbance.
3. Plot birth weight against gestation on graph in Figure 12.1.

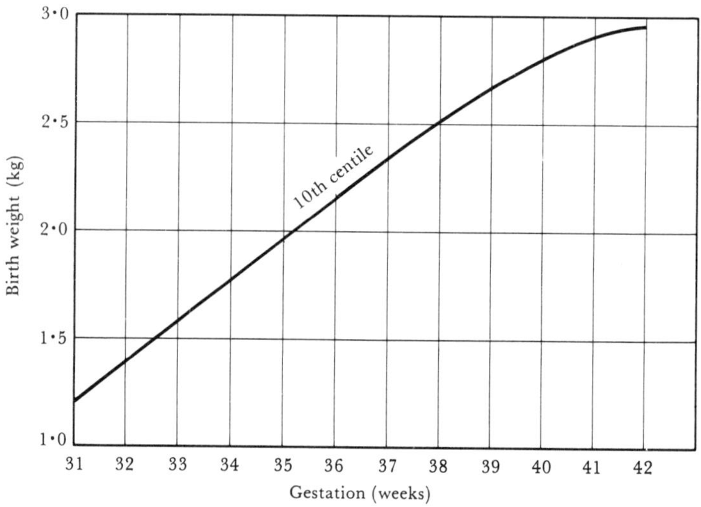

Fig 12.1 Birth weight against gentational age.

4. If baby is **preterm**, be prepared for

Hyaline membrane disease (p. 133)
Apnoeic attacks (p. 136)
Feeding difficulties
Jaundice (p. 137)

5. If baby has suffered **intra-uterine malnutrition**, be prepared for hypoglycaemia

(i) feed early (e.g. 1 h after birth)
(ii) do Dextrostix at intervals (3-12 hourly) for 48 h, and get laboratory estimation if <20 mg/100 ml
(iii) if blood glucose persistently <1.5 mmol/l or if symptoms of hypoglycaemia (convulsions, apnoea, lethargy), give dextrose infusion (p. 148).

BABIES OF DIABETIC MOTHERS

General

1. Babies of diabetic mothers who have been poorly controlled in pregnancy tend to suffer from

(i) premature birth
(ii) hyaline membrane disease (disproportionate to degree of prematurity)
(iii) hypoglycaemia.

2. They are large, plump and plethoric ('like an over-ripe tomato'), and their size and appearance may cause over-estimation of gestation.

Management

1. Assess gestation, as on p. 175, disregarding birth weight.
2. Check for hypoglycaemia above, doing Dextrostix 3 hourly for 24 hrs.
3. If any doubt about baby's ability to maintain adequate blood glucose level by oral feeds give dextrose infusion (p. 148).

HAEMORRHAGE

General

1. A baby's blood volume is c. 85 ml/kg, so a loss of only 50 ml may be a quarter of the total.
2. Blood loss may occur

   (i) through the placenta (e.g. during ante- or intra-partum haemorrhage; into a twin; in Caesarian section)
   (ii) from birth trauma (e.g. into abdomen or scalp)
   (iii) through the umbilicus (from inadequate occlusion).

Management

1. Watch for signs of hypovolaemia (pallor; hyperventilation; rising pulse, falling blood pressure).
2. Insert umbilical venous catheter (p. 177).
3. Take blood for

Hb and platelets (but Hb is no guide to loss in acute bleed)	Group
	Clotting studies

4. Give vitamin K 1 mg i.m. (if not done already).
5. Get partly-packed blood, cross-matched with mother's serum. If no time for crossmatch transfuse at once with O-ve blood c. 30 ml/kg.
6. If baby has haematemesis, check source of blood by Kleihauer test (adult haemoglobin is denatured and goes brown more readily than fetal: set up 3 tubes, with known adult blood, known fetal blood, and sample of haematemesis; dilute to same colour with water; add a few drops of 1% NaOH).

RESPIRATORY DISTRESS

General

Cardinal signs

Respiratory rate > 60/min
Sub-costal recession
Grunting or moaning expiration

Usual causes

Hyaline membrane disease (HMD)
Transient tachypnoea
Aspiration of meconium
Pneumothorax
Pneumonia
Diaphragmatic hernia

Hyaline Membrane Disease

Clinical

1. This is the commonest cause of respiratory distress and is especially associated with

Gestation <37 weeks
Birth asphyxia
Ante-partum haemorrhage
Diabetic mother

2. Signs may be present immediately after birth but sometimes do not develop for several hours. Deterioration may continue for c. 36 hours.
3. Chest x-ray may show

(i) no change
(ii) widespread granular mottling
(iii) ground glass appearance with air bronchogram.

4. There is no specific treatment: the aim is to keep the baby alive until spontaneous recovery begins.

Management

1. Minimise development of HMD in a baby at risk by

    (i) treating birth asphyxia promptly
    (ii) keeping him warm from birth onwards
    (iii) disturbing him as little as possible.

2. If it looks as though HMD may become severe and you have no special facilities, refer to a specialist unit *early* while baby is still fit to travel (see p. 148).

3. Nurse baby in an incubator with a heat shield.

4. Give oxygen (see below) in high concentration for first 6 hours then reduce to least needed to keep him pink.

5. Unless respiratory distress remains mild get chest x-ray (PA and lateral).

Oxygen therapy

A prolonged high arterial P_{O_2} in a neonate, especially if pre-term, may cause retrolental fibroplasia, while low P_{O_2} may result in brain damage. Whenever possible arterial P_{O_2} should be monitored, which is one of the main reasons for transferring babies with severe respiratory distress to a specialist unit. Where facilities and expertise are lacking, oxygen therapy must be regulated by the baby's colour.

Nutrition

1. If distress mild, feed by nasogastric tube, and nurse baby prone or on side to prevent aspiration of vomit.

2. If distress more severe, withhold oral feeds and hydrate intravenously (p. 177).

Transient Tachypnoea

1. This occurs in babies of any gestation, particularly after Casesarian section without a period of labour, and is probably due to delayed fluid clearance from the lungs.

2. Chest x-ray may show peri-hilar flaring.
3. Distress does not become serious and spontaneous recovery occurs within c. 48 hours.

Aspiration of Meconium

1. At birth if there is a possibility of aspiration of meconium intubate immediately and suck out thoroughly, even if respiration seems adequate.
2. Chest x-ray may show patchy collapse and consolidation, and often fluid in fissures.
3. Watch for pneumothorax.
4. General management as for HMD.

Pneumothorax

1. Diagnose by chest x-ray (do not be fooled by latissimus dorsi).
2. Allow to resorb by itself unless

   (i) under tension (p. 9)
   (ii) causing serious respiratory embarrassment (more likely if complicating another lung problem).

3. Give enough oxygen (see *Oxygen therapy*), p. 134) to keep the baby pink.
4. If drainage is required use neonatal chest drain or large i.v. cannula (e.g. Angiocath 14) through 4th intercostal space at mid-axillary line, and connect to underwater seal (see p. 166).

Pneumonia

1. Suspect especially after prolonged rupture of membranes, or in any baby with unexpected respiratory distress.
2. Diagnose by chest x-ray.
3. Culture

   (i) blood

(ii) gastric aspirate if baby <24 h old
(iii) CSF if any possibility of meningitis.

4. Start parenteral gentamicin and benzyl penicillin.
5. General management as for HMD.

Diaphragmatic Hernia

See p. 126.

APNOEIC ATTACKS

Diagnosis

Apnoeic attacks are usually associated with:

Prematurity
Maternal sedation
Infection (p. 144)
Hypoglycaemia
Intraventricular haemorrhage
Severe respiratory distress.

Management

1. Nurse in an incubator with

(i) an apnoea alarm
(ii) temperature not too high (may depress respiration)
(iii) as little disturbance as possible (except when he has an attack).

2. Feed small amounts 1-2 hourly (large feeds may provoke apnoea).

3. Check if mother was given opiates <6 h before delivery; if she was, give baby naloxone 0.1 mg/kg i.m.

4. Check blood glucose with Dextrostix (p. 73)

(i) if <40 mg/100 ml get laboratory estimation
(ii) if <1.75 mmol/l (c. 30 mg/100 ml) infuse 10% dextrose.

5. Terminate an attack by stimulation (e.g. flick feet or aspirate pharynx). If he has repeated attacks tie a tape round his ankle and stimulate him by tweaking it (without opening incubator).

6. If attacks are frequent and severe consider

(i) infusion with aminophylline (for dose, see p. 184)
(ii) mechanical ventilation.

JAUNDICE

General

1. Mild jaundice is very common and usually of no great importance. But jaundice may be important if

(i) it is severe enough to bring the risk of kernicterus
(ii) it indicates an underlying disorder.

2. Kernicterus most often results from Rhesus incompatibility, but can sometimes arise from other causes of jaundice. There is a risk of kernicterus if the serum bilirubin (SB) exceeds c. 350 μmol/l (c. 20 mg/100 ml), but it may occur at a lower level if the baby is

(i) preterm
(ii) hypoxic or acidotic
(iii) otherwise ill.

Clinical

1. A rough estimation of the degree of jaundice can be made by blanching the tip of the baby's nose (or the gums in a coloured baby). But this is very unreliable, especially in artifical light, and jaundice that seems more than mild should be estimated biochemically.

2. The features of kernicterus are

Early: lethargy, poor feeding, hypotonia
Late: convulsions, vomiting, spasticity

(but if these occur you are already too late).

Diagnosis

1. The commoner causes of jaundice, in approximate order of frequency, are outlined in Table 12.1.
2. Jaundice should always be investigated if

   (i) the mother is rh -ve
   (ii) it begins on the first day of life
   (iii) it appears moderate or severe, or is progressing rapidly
   (iv) the baby has other evidence of illness
   (v) it persists for more than 5 days.

Management

1. Ensure good fluid intake. If necessary

   (i) give complementary feeds of water to breast-fed baby
   (ii) tube-feed baby that will not take enough
   (iii) drip feed sick baby.

2. Check the following initially:

Mother's blood group and obstetric history	Urine for cells and reducing substances
Baby's SB, Hb, blood group, Coombs, film	Culture of urine, umbilical swab, nasal swab.

3. If diagnosis still not clear also consider

   (i) maternal haemolysins (if ABO incompatibility possible)
   (ii) culture of blood and CSF
   (iii) antibodies to rubella, toxoplasma, cytomegalovirus, herpes
   (iv) TSH

Table 12.1 Common causes of jaundice

Cause	*Usual onset (day)*	*Typical features*
'Physiological'	2 - 4	Pre-term baby; poor fluid intake
Extravasated blood	2 - 4	Bruising or haematoma
Breast milk	3 - 6	Healthy baby; jaundice may persist while breast feeding continues
Rhesus incompatibility	1 - 2	Multiparity; maternal Rh antibodies
ABO incompatibility	2 - 3	May be primipara; maternal haemolysins
Neonatal infection	2 - 14	See p. 144
Congenital infection	2 - 4	Light-for-dates baby; hepatosplenomegaly; purpura
Liver disease	2 - 14	Persisting jaundice; raised direct bilirubin
Hypothyroidism	2 - 14	Lethargy; hypotonia; large tongue
Spherocytosis	1 - 4	Family history
(Also galactosaemia, G6PD deficiency, etc)		

(v) liver function tests
(vi) G6PD test (especially in Mediterranean or Asian male infants).

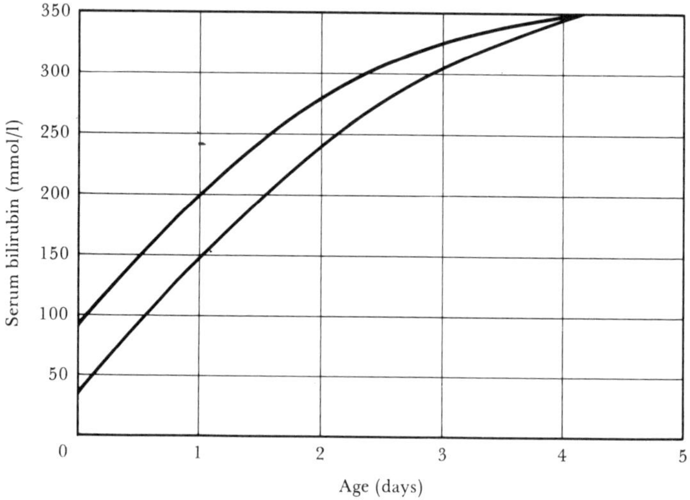

Fig 12.2 Serum bilirubin against age.

4. Plot SB against time on graph in Figure 12.2. If jaundice starts on day 1, or seems to be rising rapidly, repeat after 6 hours.

5. If SB is above or approaching lower line on the graph consider phototheraphy. Remember

(i) to cover eyes and to remove nappy
(ii) not to overheat
(iii) it may cause a harmless rash (warn mother) and loose stools.

6. If SB is above or approaching upper line on the graph transfer baby urgently for exchange transfusion.

7. Judge each baby individually, treating earlier if it is preterm, hypoxic, acidotic or ill, and later if it is full-term, large and healthy.

VOMITING

General

1. Vomiting is a very common symptom in neonates and is usually of little significance, but sometimes it may arise from one of many serious conditions.

2. A serious cause is unlikely in an otherwise healthy baby with a normal weight pattern (a loss of 10% in the first week is acceptable).

3. Features that particularly suggest a more serious cause are

(i) an ill or dehydrated baby
(ii) abdominal distension and failure to pass meconium or changing stools
(iii) bile in the vomit (bile is dark green not yellow)
(iv) concomitant diarrhoea.

Diagnosis

1. More common and not usually serious causes are outlined in Table 12.2.

2. Less common, but more serious causes are set out in Table 12.3.

3. Other causes are featured in Table 12.4.

Table 12.2 Common causes of vomiting

Condition	*Typical features*
Mucus gastritis	First 2 days of life; may improve after stomach washout
Cerebral irritation	Precipitate or difficult delivery; first 4 days of life
Wind	Poor feeding and winding technique; belches with vomit
Incompetent cardia	Worse when laid down; may persist for months

Table 12.3 Serious causes of vomiting

Obstruction	*Typical features*	*Tests*
Pyloric stenosis	No bile staining; unusual in first 10 days; projectile vomits; visible peristalsis; worried baby	Test feed → palpable tumour Serum $Cl^- \downarrow$ $HCO_3^- \uparrow$
Duodenal atresia	Hydramnios; vomiting starts early, usually bile-stained	X-ray → double bubble
Meconium ileus	Family history of cystic fibrosis; distension; no passage of meconium	X-ray → fluid levels, mottled bowel shadow
Inguinal hernia	Mass in groin or scrotum	
Volvulus	Abdominal mass; bloody stool	X-ray → dilated loop
Hirschsprung's	Family history; distension; constipation relieved by rectal examination	Manometry Rectal biopsy

Management

1. Nurse baby on side or prone to reduce risk of aspiration.
2. Make sure you see a specimen of vomit.
3. Record all feeds, vomits, stools, urine and daily weights.
4. Check for features detailed above and do relevant tests.
5. At first sign of dehydration start i.v. fluids.
6. If you suspect obstruction

Table 12.4 Various causes of vomiting

Causes	*Typical features*	*Tests*
Infection		
Gastroenteritis	Diarrhoea	Stool culture
Meningitis	Convulsions; lethargy; apnoeic attacks	Lumbar puncture
Pyelonephritis	Ill baby	Urine microscopy and culture
Necrotising enterocolitis	Distended abdomen; bloody stools	X-ray → dilated loops; intramural gas
Metabolic disturbance		
Adrenal hyperplasia	Family history; abnormal genitalia	Serum Na^{+}↓, urine Na^{+}↑
Hypoglycaemia	Light-for-dates baby; convulsions; lethargy	Blood glucose
Galactosaemia	Jaundice	Clinitest of urine
Miscellaneous		
Subdural haematoma	Difficult delivery; bulging fontanelle; convulsions	Subdural taps (see p. 173)
Cardiac failure	Hepatomegaly; tachycardia (see also p. 16)	Chest x-ray, ECG

(i) put down nasogastric tube, aspirate stomach contents and leave on free drainage
(ii) hydrate i.v.
(iii) take blood for Hb, electrolytes and urea, and group.
(iv) get surgical advice *early*.

INFECTION

General

1. Infection is especially likely when

   (i) there has been prolonged rupture of membranes or protracted labour
   (ii) the baby has a low birth weight, a malformation, or another illness
   (iii) the umbilical vessels have been catheterised
   (iv) the baby has been intubated for more than a brief period.

2. A wide variety of organisms may cause neonatal infection, the most usual being coliforms, *Staph. aureus* and Group B *Streptococcus*.

3. There is often bacteraemia and spread to more than one system.

4. Untreated infection can quickly overwhelm a neonate, so antibiotics often have to be started before proof is obtained.

Diagnosis

1. The onset may be insidious, with only vague and non-specific indications, e.g.

- Lethargy, poor feeding and failure to gain weight
- Poor colour (pallor, cyanosis, mottling)
- Slightly raised or slightly lowered temperature
- Irritability and sometimes convulsions
- Vomiting or mild diarrhoea
- Late or persistent jaundice
- Tachypnoea or apnoeic attacks
- Persistent tachycardia.

2. Sometimes there may be more specific signs, e.g.

Septicaemia.	Rash, splenomegaly
Meningitis.	Specific signs are unhelpful: a bulging fontanelle occurs late, and neck rigidity is unusual
Pneumonia.	Rapid respiration, flaring alae nasi, chest signs
Osteitis.	Swelling, pseudo-paresis
Urinary tract.	Cells and protein in urine
Intestinal tract.	Profuse or bloody diarrhoea
Superficial.	Skin, eyes, nails, scalp, umbilicus (these may be associated with deeper infection).

Management

1. Regardless of the signs do all these tests:

Chest x-ray
Swabs from nose, throat, ear, umbilicus and any superficial lesions
Blood culture (two bottles if possible)
Lumbar puncture (get a Gram stain and culture regardless of the cell count)
Urine culture (if necessary by supra-pubic aspiration)
Stool culture (or rectal swab).

2. Find out if mother has any signs of infection, especially infected lochia, and check any cultures taken from her.

3. If infection seems likely but organism cannot be immediately identified, as soon as cultures have been taken start treatment with gentamicin and benzyl penicillin (for dosage see p. 185). Modify antibiotics in light of culture results and continue for at least 5 days.

4. If CSF results suggest meningitis add chloramphenicol to above (good penetration of blood/brain barrier).

5. If necrotising enterocolitis, add i.v. metronidazole (for anaerobes).

6. Intensify precautions against cross-infection (especially hand-washing), and watch adjacent babies carefully.

CONVULSIONS

General

1. Seizures are fairly common in neonates, but typical grand mal convulsions are unusual. Seizures usually take the form of

(i) focal twitching
(ii) generalised tonic spasm, often with apnoea.

2. Seizures which begin in the first 3 days are more often associated with brain damage and have a worse prognosis than those beginning later.

Diagnosis

1. There are numerous causes, the more common are set out in Table 12.5.

2. If cause is not clear do these tests:

Blood glucose (plus immediate Dextrostix)	Urine sugars (Clinitest)
	Lumbar puncture (p. 162)
Serum Na^+, Ca^{++}, Mg^{++}	Skull transillumination.

3. Consider also these tests:

Serum bilirubin	Subdural taps (p. 173)
Urine amino acids	Pyridoxine 25 mg i.v.
Specific IgM (for congenital infection)	EEG (usually more help for prognosis than diagnosis).
Skull x-ray	

Table 12.5 Common causes of convulsions

Condition	*Usual onset*	*Typical features*
Congenital malformation	Birth - day 2	Other CNS abnormalities
Birth trauma	Birth - day 2	History
Perinatal asphyxia	Birth - day 2	History
Congenital infection	Birth onwards	Light-for-dates; hepatosplenomegaly; purpura
Inborn errors of metabolism	Birth onwards	Family history; hepatomegaly
Hypoglycaemia	Birth - day 3	Light-for-dates or post-term; diabetic mother; apnoea; lethargy
Intraventricular haemorrhage	Day 1 - 3	Pre-term; severe respiratory distress
Hypocalcaemia (or hypomagnesaemia)	Day 5 - 10	Active but jittery baby; feeding with high phosphate milk
Meningitis	Any time	Ill baby; vomiting; lethargy

Management

1. If respiration inadequate give 100% oxygen by mask.
2. Terminate fit in progress (unless it consists of only minimal twitching) with

   (i) diazepam i.v. (but do not give so much as to depress respiration)

or

   (ii) paraldehyde i.m.

3. If fits keep recurring start phenobarbitone.
4. If **hypoglycaemia**

   (i) give immediate i.v. dextrose 20% 5 ml/kg (preferably by peripheral vein)

then

   (ii) give oral feeds every hour, and/or give i.v. infusion of dextrose 10% (up to rate for daily need – p. 181).
   (iii) monitor blood glucose with Dextrostix (hourly at first) to maintain level of >2.5 mmol/l.

5. If **hypocalcaemia:**

   (i) give slow i.v. infusion of calcium gluconate 10% 0.2 ml/kg and magnesium sulphate 50% 0.1 ml/kg
   (ii) change to low phosphate milk (breast milk, SMA *Gold Cap*, Cow and Gate *Premium*, Ostermilk *Complete*)
   (iii) add calcium gluconate 100 mg/kg to feeds 6 hourly.

6. If **meningitis**, see p. 145.

TRANSPORT

Transfer of sick baby

If a sick baby has to be transferred to another hospital

1. Tell parents what is happening and make sure mother sees baby before transfer. If possible arrange for mother to be transferred too.

2. Transfer as soon as any immediate resuscitation has been completed. If you wait he may deteriorate and become too sick to travel.

3. Ensure that a doctor experienced in neonatal resuscitation travels in the ambulance. He should take with him

A full perinatal history
A sample of mother's blood
Consent for operation (where appropriate)
Equipment for resuscitation

4. Keep the baby warm by

   (i) wrapping him in a silver swaddler lined with gamgee
   (ii) putting him in a pre-heated incubator or in a cot warmed by hot-water bottles (take care not to burn his skin).

5. If the baby has respiratory distress intubate before transfer and give IPPV by hand or machine *en route*, using 100% oxygen.
6. If he has an umbilical drip which is not essential on journey disconnect it and leave the sealed end *in situ*.
7. If possible monitor heart rate with a machine (auscultation and palpation are almost impossible while travelling).
8. Leave baby's face visible for observation of colour and if necessary give oxygen in high concentration by mask.
9. If urgent procedures are necessary *en route*, ask the driver to stop.
10. If you have to go by crowded roads, ask for a police escort.

13 Procedures

VENEPUNCTURE

General

1. Before you begin ask yourself

   (i) is a blood sample *really* necessary?
   (ii) are there any other blood tests to be done which you can include in the same venepuncture?
   (iii) if i.v. drugs are to be given can you inject through the same needle?

2. Never try to take blood from a moving target. It is safer and often kinder to have the child held firmly, so make sure you have a capable nurse to help you (or two nurses if need be).
3. If child is particularly scared consider

   (i) sedation in advance
   (ii) spraying skin at puncture site with ethyl chloride.

4. Don't say 'it won't hurt' because it always does and he'll never trust doctors again.
5. A small sample can be obtained by pricking pulp of a finger or lobe of an ear (or heel of an infant), though this may be more painful than a good venepuncture.
6. If taking blood from the periphery, you can encourage vasodilatation by warming whole child with extra blankets and clothes, or the limb with warm water or towels.
7. If possible occlude the vein proximally with a tourniquet, which is more effective than someone's grasp.
8. Pay particular attention to the needle:

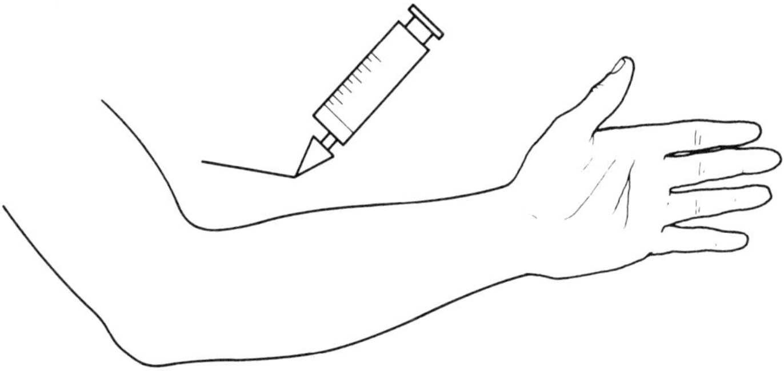

Fig 13.1 Needle bent for venepuncture

(i) you may get a better angle of approach by bending it slightly (Fig. 13.1)
(ii) sometimes a butterfly (Abbot) may be easier (e.g. for a large sample from a wriggly child)
(iii) in a baby a No. 23 needle is large enough, filled with heparin to reduce clotting (unless the test will be affected, e.g. prothrombin time)
(iv) consider using an in-dwelling needle if another sample will be needed soon; leave it firmly secured and filled with heparin.

9. Before you start check

(i) needle is firmly on syringe
(ii) barrel of syringe is not stuck
(iii) all the right tubes are at hand
(iv) blood-culture bottles are not ice-cold.

10. When using a small vein do not suck too hard or vein will collapse. Be patient and you may go on getting blood intermittently for some time (but with increasing likelihood of clotting and of distortion of serum K^+ by haemolysis).

Veins

The choice will depend on

- Age and condition of child
- Amount of blood required
- Relative risks of sites available
- Your preference and experience
- Need to preserve veins for drips.

For various sites, see Table 13.1.

Notes on sites

Hand, wrist, foot. Warming often helpful.

Wrist. More painful.

Ante-cubital fossa. Go for vein you can feel rather than vein you can see; distinguish brachial artery (but if you get into it accidentally

Table 13.1 Various sites for venepuncture

Site	*Age of child*	*Amount of blood*	*Suitability for drip*	*Risk*
Back of hand	Any	+++	++	–
Flexor surface of wrist	Any	+	–	–
Ante-cubital fossa	Any	++++	+	–
Dorsum of foot	Any	+	+	–
External jugular	0 – 4 years	++	–	+
Scalp	0 – 2 years	+	++	–
Femoral	Any	+++++	–	+
Internal jugular	0 – 4 years	+++++	–	++

you might as well take your blood, applying longer pressure afterwards).

External jugular, scalp. Have child help firmly with head tilted slightly down (and turned to opposite side for jugular); crying makes the veins more prominent; afterwards sit child up immediately.

Femoral. The sequence of structures, medial to lateral, is vein-artery-nerve; have child held firmly with hip abducted c. 40° and not quite fully extended; clean skin thoroughly and feel for artery; go in vertically downwards just medial to artery and just below inguinal ligament to depth just short of bone; apply suction and withdraw needle slowly, holding it still as soon as blood flows; if you hit artery you might as well take your blood, applying longer pressure afterwards; sometimes in a baby artery goes into spasm and leg becomes horribly blue, in which case keep it warm and observe closely till it returns to normal; the other main risk is to hit bone and cause osteitis.

Internal jugular. Relatively safe in the hands of experts but too risky for the unsupervised beginner so not described here.

ARTERIAL PUNCTURE

General

1. See points 2, 3 and 4 under *Venepuncture* (p. 150).
2. You only need arterial blood for estimation of P_{O_2} (P_{CO_2} and pH can be estimated from an arterialised capillary sample).
3. Before you start consider if you can take any other necessary blood samples through same needle.
4. If you are going to need repeated samples consider inserting cannula.
5. A No. 23 needle is big enough. Fill dead space with heparin.

6. Try not to change ambient P_{O_2} during procedure (e.g. take child's arm out of tent rather than opening up tent completely).

7. Arteries are more elusive than veins and require firmer anchoring.

8. It is sometimes hard to be certain whether you have got arterial or venous blood, though colour and ease of flow may be helpful. If in doubt send for estimation anyway; the results may help you decide, and the P_{CO_2} and pH from a central vein will give a rough guide to arterial values.

9. After puncture see that pressure is applied for at least 5 min and then check that bleeding has completely stopped.

Sites

Radial artery. Lies just under skin in middle of groove between styloid process of radius and tendon of flexor carpi radialis; has advantages of an alternative supply (ulnar artery) and natural anchoring: do not extend wrist but keep hand in line with forearm; go in at 45° with bevel of needle upwards at proximal skin crease of wrist; if you do not get blood just underneath skin, go deeper till you just touch bone and try again on way back.

Brachial artery. Medial side of antecubital fossa; very mobile.

Femoral artery. Biggest but most hazardous; be extra diligent over haemostasis.

Temporal artery. Possible even in neonates; artery runs just anterior to pinna.

INTRAVENOUS INFUSION

General

1. See points 2, 3, 4, 6 and 7 under *Venepuncture* (p. 150).

2. Be calm and unhurried (a cup of coffee beforehand often helps).

Choice of needle

A butterfly (Abbot) is the easier to insert, but seldom lasts more than 48 hours and being rigid may be more readily dislodged at an unstable site. With practice a small flexible cannula (e.g. Longdwell No. 23) can be put into almost any vein that would take a butterfly and will usually last longer.

Size of needle

Use largest size that vein will comfortably accept. An infusion pump is very helpful, especially with small needles, both to ensure correct rate and to reduce clotting. Blood, particularly packed cells, seldom runs properly through a needle less than size 21 without a pump.

Sites

Back of hand. Usually the most convenient for all ages but may not be possible in a chubby baby.

Ante-cubital fossa. Allows a bigger needle but is more cumbersome because of the joint.

Radial aspect of forearm. May be suitable in older children but not usually in babies.

Dorsum of foot. Convenient but veins are usually small.

Scalp. Usually possible up to c. 24 months; the best veins run down towards ears or near middle of forehead; choose straight segment of vein, aiming to enter it at end nearest vertex; easier to cannulate than you might expect and will usually take a No. 23 Longdwell; shave as little of scalp as possible; always warn the mother.

Technique

Most people develop their own technique and it is best to use the method you feel most confident with. These notes describe a method of inserting a cannula such as a Longdwell.

1. Make sure you have the following ready at hand:

Razor.
Scalpel blade.
Gauze swab.
Cannula (check that it slides easily on the needle, and remove stopper).
Drip set, with fine tubing extension added, ready run through.
Small syringe filled with saline.
Sticking tape cut to suitable lengths.
Appropriate splint (2 spatulae wrapped in tape will often do for baby).

2. Ensure child is held firmly but comfortably, and be comfortable yourself.
3. Shave hair from over puncture site and where you plan to stick tape (but not more than you need to).
4. Cleanse area thoroughly.
5. Make sure vein is occluded proximally (by a tourniquet on limb or by a nurse's finger on scalp).
6. Make a 2 mm incision through skin just before point where you plan to enter vein, taking care not to puncture vein itself (this is to avoid distorting small cannula by forcing it through skin).
7. Wipe away any blood with swab and insert point of needle and cannula through incision.
8. With your left hand hold skin tense enough to keep vein straight and steady, but no so tight as to empty it.
9. Advance needle briskly into the vein and pause.
10. If a back-flow of blood appears you are probably in. If it does not, try rotating the needle. If that does not work, try another brisk advance.

11. If you have advanced along the whole segment of vein without success, draw back and try again. But once a haematoma has appeared your chances of success are almost nil.

12. Once you think you are in vein, gently ease needle in another 2 mm, slide cannula down over needle and withdraw needle (this can be a tricky manoeuvre especially in a wriggly child; practise doing it with one hand so that your other hand can continue to help steady the target); if you are in vein the cannula will slide in easily and painlessly; push it as far as it will comfortably go.

13. If you are still not sure that you are in vein or if end of cannula seems to be blocked, syringe a little saline through.

14. Secure drip as in Figure 13.2. This method is suitable for scalp or limb, is flexible and allows easy inspection.

15. On a limb, a splint will usually be needed to give stability and the site may need to be protected by a bandage.

16. A small child's hands will usually have to be restrained to stop him pulling the drip out.

17. If you fail more than twice ask someone else to help before all veins are ruined.

VENOUS CUTDOWN

General

1. Avoid venous cutdown, if possible. It should only be necessary when

(i) infusion is urgent and peripheral veins are collapsed (e.g. haemorrhage or severe gastro-enteritis)
(ii) all possible percutaneous drip sites are used up.

2. The long saphenous vein at the ankle is usually the most convenient, though the cephalic and basilic veins at the elbow are also possible.

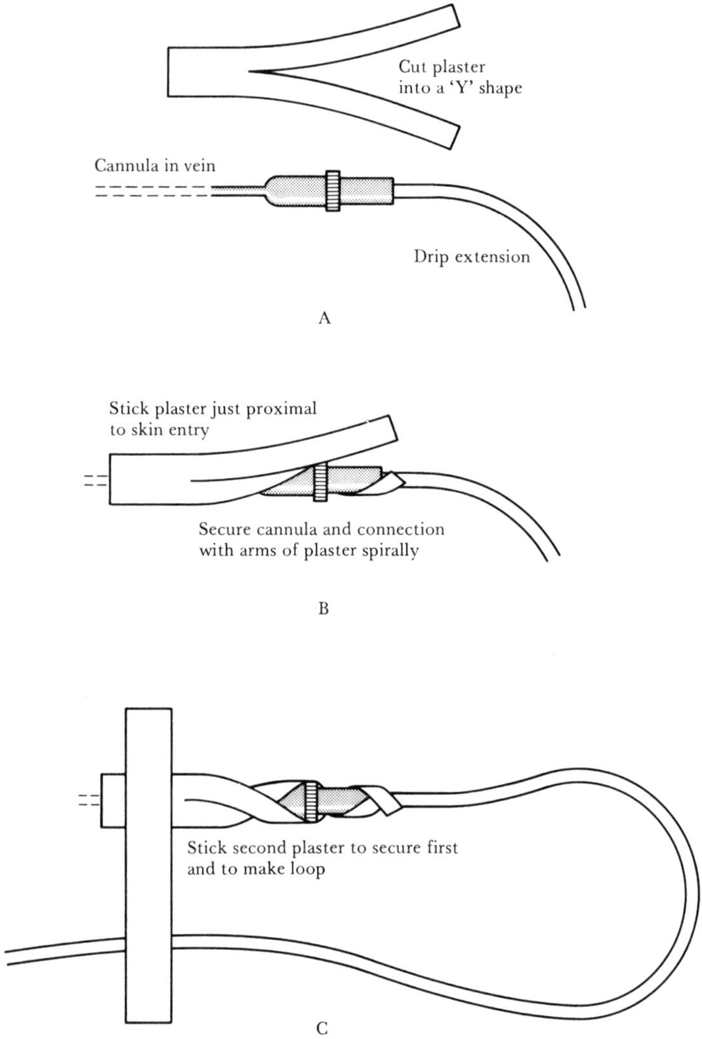

Fig 13.2 Method of securing intravenous cannula.

3. Sedate child in advance if possible.
4. Be sure you have

   (i) really good lighting
   (ii) a target kept completely still by splinting and by capable nurses.

5. Be scrupulous about sterility.
6. Check that you have the following ready:

Cleansing fluid
Local anaesthetic.
Scalpel.
Mosquito artery forceps and small dissecting forceps (both of paediatric size).
Very fine-pointed scissors.
Fine dilator.
Catheter (size 21) with rounded end.
Syringe filled with saline.
Fine catgut.
Silk stitch (with needle).
Drip set with fine tubing extension ready run through.
Antibiotic spray.
Small sterile dressing.
Plaster strapping.

Technique (for long saphenous cut-down)

1. The vein runs upwards and slightly posteriorly over the anterior part of the medial malleolus (Fig. 13.3). The site for the incision is at the upper margin of the malleolus, at right angles to the vein and so at about 15° to the horizontal (the posterior end being lower).

2. Cleanse skin thoroughly, and infiltrate incision line, and 2 cm below it, with local anaesthetic.

3. Make skin incision, *not more than 2 cm long*.

4. Identify and separate the vein (there are no other superficial structures except cutaneous nerves at this point).

5. Pass under it a loop of catgut; cut loop to make two lengths, and work them to each end of exposed stretch of vein (Fig. 13.4); tie distal catgut leaving ends long, but leave proximal catgut untied.

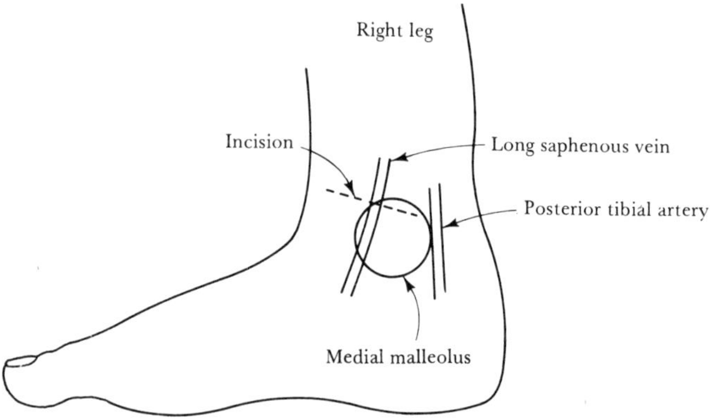

Fig 13.3 Medial aspect of ankle showing site for long saphenous cutdown.

6. Attach catheter to syringe and fill it with saline.
7. Keeping vein steady and straight by holding distal catgut in your left hand, with fine scissors make a 1 mm nick in top surface of vein in middle of exposed stretch.
8. Hold catheter with forceps and introduce it into lumen of vein. If this proves difficult

(i) check that your nick has in fact penetrated to lumen and that you are not in wall
(ii) try dilating lumen gently with dilator.

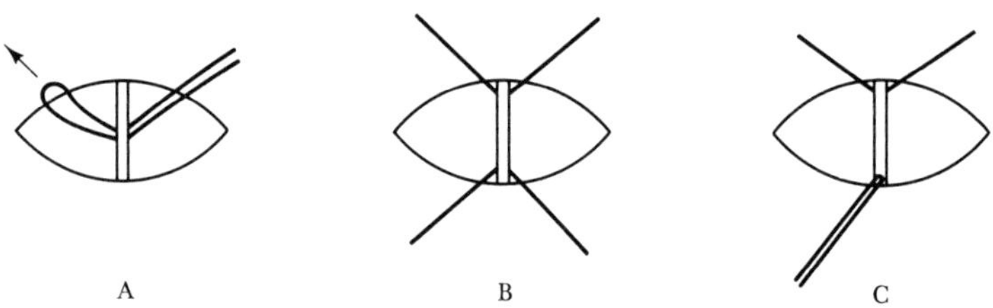

Fig 13.4 Method of passing cat-gut beneath vein.

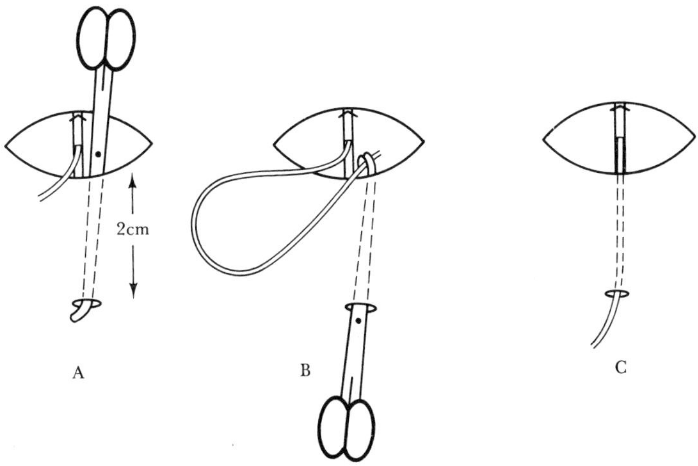

Fig 13.5 Mosquito forceps making subcutaneous tunnel for catheter.

9. Slide catheter as far up vein as it will easily go; check that there is free flow through it by injecting a little saline; secure it by tying proximal catgut; cut all ends fairly short.

10. With mosquito forceps make a subcutaneous tunnel for 2 cm downwards from incision, and expose tip of forceps with a nick in overlying skin (Fig. 13.5).

11. Extract forceps and then insert tip from the outside through nick and back up subcutaneous tunnel; grasp end of catheter and pull it down through tunnel and out through skin.

(Steps 10 and 11 are not essential but reduce risk of infection and allow quicker healing and less scarring.)

12. Connect up catheter to drip set.

13. Sew up main incision carefully with silk. Spray area with antibiotic spray and put sterile dressing over catheter exit.

14. Secure drip tubing with plaster, making a loop in tube to prevent catheter being pulled straight out by accident.

LUMBAR PUNCTURE

General

1. Usually easier in a child than in an adult because spine is more readily flexed and ligaments are softer.

2. Success depends as much on the nurse as the doctor. Be sure you have one or more experienced nurses to hold the child: even if he is lying still to start with he is bound to move when you begin. Never try to LP a moving target.

3. Always sedate an older child (e.g. >3 years) unless there is a very good reason not to. A useful technique is to take blood samples with a butterfly needle and inject back through the same needle a sedative/analgesic such as pentazocine.

4. Use local anaesthetic in an older child, but omit it in a baby because it may obscure the anatomical landmarks.

5. Be sure you have all the equipment and sample bottles at hand before you start.

6. Ask yourself again: could this child have raised intracranial pressure? Go by history as much as by papilloedema, which may not have had time to develop.

Method

1. Child should be positioned lying on his left side curled up into a ball with spine as well flexed as possible; his lumbar spine should be right at edge of bed with coronal and horizontal planes exactly vertical (this posture is very uncomfortable, especially if he has meningism, so do not get him there till you are completely ready).

2. Scrub and glove up, and check equipment, in particular that

(i) needle is right size (e.g. size 21 for larger children, 23 for babies) and has stilette which is of right length and not stuck

(ii) tops of sample bottles are loosened
(iii) manometer (if applicable) connects properly
(iv) local anaesthetic is drawn up into small syringe with very fine needle.

3. Clean target area with spirit and cover the surrounds, including iliac crest, with sterile drapes or paper.

4. L3/4 is the most suitable interspinous space and will be found perpendicularly below iliac crest (L2/3 and L4/5 can also be used).

5. Except in a baby infiltrate overlying skin with a little local anaesthetic, using very fine needle. Pause for 30 sec, then infiltrate deeper.

6. Get child curled tightly now.

7. With stilette in place and bevel pointing towards the head, insert needle in mid-line halfway between the spinous processes, exactly horizontal and aimed towards umbilicus.

8. Push in gently, frequently checking that it remains horizontal, and withdrawing stilette at intervals to see if fluid emerges.

9. There should be a drop in resistance as needle enters theca. When you feel this withdraw stilette. If no fluid flows, try rotating it. If still no fluid flows, try replacing stilette and advancing needle a fraction more.

10. If you hit bone before you reach the theca, partly withdraw needle, check your alignment, and re-insert with appropriate shift of direction.

11. If frank blood emerges you have probably transversed theca and entering the plexus of veins beyond it. Withdraw completely from that site, and try again in adjacent space.

12. It is not usually worth attempting to measure the pressure in a crying child, but you should attempt to do so if it seems relevant. Get an assistant to steady upper end of manometer, and then to save fluid in it by putting finger over top.

13. After withdrawing needle immediately unflex child's back so as to seal off needle track. Put a small plaster over puncture site. There is no need to use collodion, which makes a sticky mess.

14. If you have not made a successful tap after 15 min ask someone else to try.

Tests on CSF

1. You can safely take 10 ml of fluid. Collect it in successive tubes and if suspecting meningitis send for

Always
Cell count (on final tube)
Bacterial culture
Gram stain

When cells present
Counter-immunoelectrophoresis (if available)
Estimation of protein and glucose

When appropriate
Viral culture
Stain and culture for AFB

2. Save a little fluid to examine under microscope yourself. Do not try and assess it just by holding it up to the light; infected CSF can sometimes look 'gin-clear'.
3. If you can only get a drop or two of fluid, send it for culture anyway.
4. If tap is traumatic and the fluid blood-stained, get the cells counted and compare ratio of red to white cells with that in peripheral blood.

MOUTH-TO-MOUTH VENTILATION

General

1. This method, properly used, can keep a child with respiratory arrest alive for several hours. Start it at once rather than

Table 13.2 Lung volumes (approx)

Age	*Vital capacity*	*% adult VC*
5 years	1.2 litres	25%
8 years	2.5 litres	55%
16 years	4 litres	90%

waiting for equipment to arrive.

2. There is enough oxygen in the air you exhale to sustain life; the first portion you exhale, being from your dead space, is not deoxygenated at all.

Method

1. Lay child on his side and clear any vomit from his mouth and pharynx.
2. Then lay him on his back with neck in a neutral position.
3. Insert an airway (if available).
4. With one hand occlude his nostrils, and with other hold jaw up and monitor carotid pulse.
5. Put your mouth over the child's, at right angles.
6. Get someone to press gently on the thyroid cartilage so as to occlude oesophagus (or do it yourself with little finger of hand with which you are holding jaw).
7. Inflate child's lungs so that the chest expands visibly, but do not blow in too much air for his size.
8. Approximate lung volumes are outlined in Table 13.2.
9. Remove your mouth to allow elastic recoil of his lungs to expel the breath. Keep up a rate of c. 20 breaths/min.

Babies

The same principles apply, but with the following modifications:

1. Cover his nose as well as his mouth with your mouth.
2. Use only the air from your puffed out cheeks, not from your lungs, otherwise you may rupture his lungs.

CHEST DRAIN

(These notes are for pneumothorax, but are applicable with modification to haemothorax)

General

1. The best sites are
   - (i) in 2nd intercostal space in mid-clavicular line (easier to get at)
   - (ii) in c. 4th intercostal space in mid-axillary line (usually more comfortable for child).
2. The vessels and nerves run just under each rib, so make your incision in lower part of intercostal space.
3. Use a big enough tube; too small a tube may get blocked. A rough guide is given in Table 13.3.

Table 13.3 Guide to size of tube for chest drainage

Age	*Tube*
<6 months	Argyle 12 (or Angiocath 14)
6 months - 2 years	Argyle 11
2 - 6 years	Argyle 10
6 - 12 years	Argyle 9
>12 years	Argyle 8

Method

1. Check physical signs and chest x-ray.
2. Observe full sterile technique and wear gloves.
3. Make sure all equipment is ready and that tubing connects up properly. Minimum equipment is as follows:

Cleansing fluid	Silk stitch (with needle)
Connective tubing	Trochar and catheter
Local anaesthetic	Antibiotic spray
Underwater seal	Large pair of forceps
Fine-bladed scalpel	Plaster strapping

4. Position child lying back at 45° for site 1, and leaning forwards on to pillows for site 2.
5. Clean skin thoroughly.
6. Infiltrate skin overlying site with local anaesthetic using very fine needle, then change to larger needle and infiltrate right down to pleura.
7. Incise skin and underlying fascia.
8. Insert loose purse-string suture round incision.
9. Push in trochar and catheter (you may have to push quite hard so keep a finger 2 cm from the point to act as a stop if it goes in suddenly).
10. Insert 6-12 cm (according to child's age) of catheter into pleural space, aiming to position the end at apex of lung.
11. Extract trochar and clamp off distal part of catheter with forceps.
12. Pull purse-string tight and tie it round catheter so as to anchor it.
13. Connect up catheter to underwater seal and remove forceps.
14. Ask an older child to cough, which should expel air. With a small child the fluid level in the tubing does not move much with respiration.
15. Spray incision with antibiotic and anchor catheter more securely with plaster strapping.
16. Get chest x-ray to check catheter's position and effect.

Emergency Method

If there is no proper equipment at hand, do as follows:

1. Insert a large intravenous needle and cannula (e.g. Angiocath 14).
2. Extract needle and connect cannula to a drip set.
3. Cut off the drip set tubing just below the reservoir and immerse cut end in sterile water below chest level to act as a seal.

INTUBATION

General

1. If you are not confident of your ability to intubate a child get some practice in theatre *soon*: you never know when you may have to cope with an emergency by yourself.
2. The technique is the same as in adults and is usually easier (unless there is swelling in as in epiglottitis).
3. Familiarise yourself in advance with the emergency equipment on every ward you cover, in particular making sure that

   (i) laryngoscopes work
   (ii) endotracheal tubes are right size
   (iii) connections all fit.

4. If a child needs intubating send for an anaesthetist at once. If situation is not too urgent wait till he comes and get it done expertly. But if necessary press on yourself and when he arrives get him to check what you have done.
5. Do not try to intubate a struggling child. If he is able to struggle he probably does not require emergency intubation and it is usually better to wait for an anaesthetist.

Technique

1. Lay child on his back and remove head of bed to give clear access; if it is not removable turn child round or put him on floor.
2. Get someone to give 100% oxygen by bag and mask while you are getting ready.
3. Have a sucker ready to remove mucus or vomit.
4. Select an ET tube and lubricate it lightly with jelly. The diameter of this tube should be

   (i) about the same as child's little finger
   (ii) just able to fit inside child's nostril
   (iii) roughly according to the scale in Table 13.4.

5. Stand behind child's head, put a rolled towel under his neck and extend atlanto-occipital joint.
6. Inflate lungs 2 or 3 times thoroughly with 100% oxygen by bag and mask.
7. Holding laryngoscope in left hand slide blade over tongue until tip rests in groove between tongue and epiglottis (Fig. 13.6).
8. Take care not to squeeze lips against teeth or pivot laryngoscope on upper teeth.

Table 13.4 Guide to size of tube for intubation

Age		*Diameter (mm)*
neonate	small	3.0
	normal	3.5
2 years		4
5 years		5
7 years		6
10 years		7
14 years		8

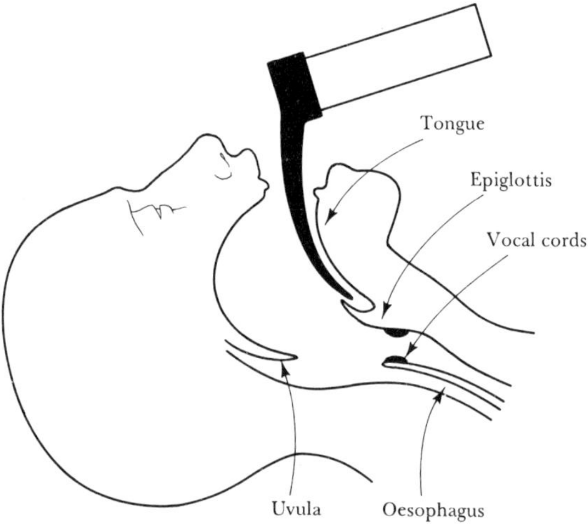

Fig 13.6 Insertion of laryngoscope for intubation

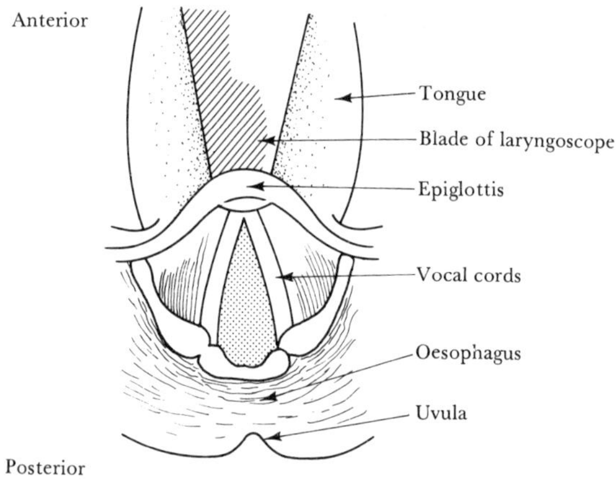

Fig 13.7 View down larynx as seen by intubator

9. Suck out any mucus or vomit as you progress.

10. Lift laryngoscope slightly upwards, compressing root of tongue and raising epiglottis. The vocal cords should then come into view (Fig. 13.7).

11. If you cannot see cords get someone to press on thyroid cartilage; this should push larynx backwards and into view (but will not compress it because it is rigid).

12. Holding ET tube in right hand insert tip between cords, going about 1 cm beyond in a baby and about 2 cm beyond in a larger child.

13. If cords are in spasm wait until they relax: hypoxia will eventually make them do so.

14. If you have not succeeded after 1 min, resume inflation by bag and mask for 2 min before trying again.

15. If you can see cords but shape of larynx prevents you manipulating end of tube between them, try using an introducer, which you should first bend to shape you need.

16. Once you are in, check that air is entering both sides of chest. If air is entering only one side, you are probably in a bronchus and should try withdrawing a little.

17. Once in position, inflate and clamp cuff (if cuffed tube), and secure tube at angle of mouth with tape twisted round tube and tied round head.

LARYNGOSTOMY

General

1. Always try and avoid an emergency by referring *early* to anaesthetist or ENT surgeon any child who is likely to develop serious respiratory obstruction (e.g. trauma to mouth, epiglottitis).

2. Prefer intubation to surgical methods whenever possible.

3. If intubation is not possible and there is total respiratory

obstruction, laryngostomy will provide an adequate airway until expert help arrives.

4. Laryngostomy is preferable to emergency tracheostomy, which is very hazardous and takes longer.

Method

1. The only essential equipment is

either

(i) a scalpel and laryngostomy tube (preferably)

or

(ii) a scalpel only

or

(iii) a wide-bore needle (e.g. Angiocath 14).

2. Lie child on his back and extend neck.
3. Locate cricothyroid membrane between thyroid and cricoid cartilages (Figure 13.8).
4. *Either*

(i) with a scalpel make small vertical incision through skin and then through the membrane, nearer the lower than

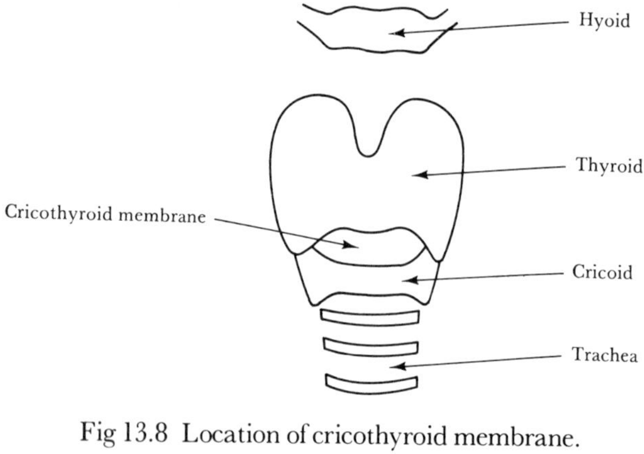

Fig 13.8 Location of cricothyroid membrane.

the upper cartilage (an artery runs along lower border of thyroid cartilage); insert laryngostomy tube

or

(ii) make incision as above; insert handle of scalpel through incision and rotate it through 90° to maintain an opening

or

(iii) insert the needle with bevel downwards in midline, aiming slightly downwards, through the skin and the membrane and into lumen of larynx.

5. Suck out blood or secretions with a fine catheter passed through the aperture.
6. Apply 100% oxygen to the aperture by tube or funnel.
7. If child has stopped breathing, inflate lungs by blowing down needle or by applying your mouth over incision.

SUBDURAL TAPS

General

1. Subdural taps are possible only in children whose sutures have not yet fused (in older children they can be done through a burr hole).
2. They are made at least 3 cm from the midline, either at the lateral angles of the anterior fontanelle or in the coronal suture beyond (Fig. 13.9).
3. Subdural collections are often bilateral so always tap both sides.
4. Observe scrupulous aseptic technique.

Method

1. Have child wrapped in sheet and placed on firm surface.

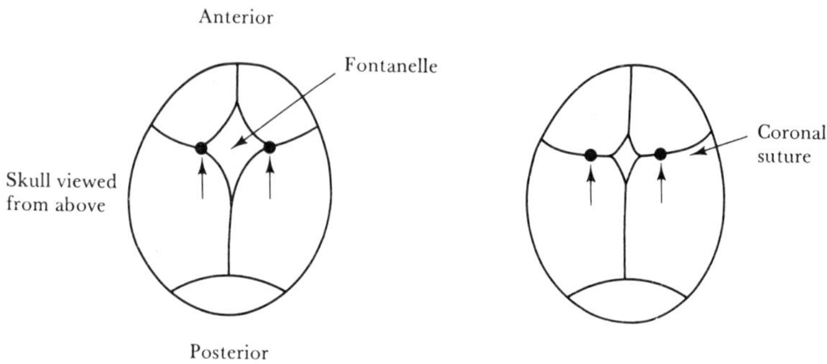

Fig 13.9 Sites for subdural taps.

2. Shave site and clean skin thoroughly.
3. Using very fine needle infiltrate with local anaesthetic.
4. Pull skin tightly to one side (to make Z track) and insert subdural needle perpendicularly to skull to depth of c. 5 mm, gripping shaft of needle firmly to prevent its going in suddenly and penetrating too deep.
5. Remove stilette and see if fluid emerges, rotating needle by 90° stages through 360°. If nothing emerges after 30 secs go 5 mm further and try again.
6. Subdural fluid is usually bloody, brown or straw-coloured, and always has a very high protein content (get this measured if distinction from CSF is needed).
7. If subdural fluid emerges freely do not drain more than 30 ml from one side before tapping the other in case unequal pressure makes brain shift. Never suck fluid out with syringe.
8. When needle is withdrawn a little fluid often oozes out (though Z track should reduce this).
9. Always send a sample for culture.

ASSESSMENT OF GESTATIONAL AGE

Score the following four factors, and apply total score to Table 13.5. The accuracy of this method is ± 2 weeks.

Skin texture

Tested by picking up a fold of abdominal skin between finger and thumb, and by inspection.

0 very thin with a gelatinous feel
1 thin and smooth
2 smooth and of medium thickness; irritation rash and superficial peeling may be present
3 slight thickening and stiff feeling with superficial cracking and peeling especially evident on the hands and feet
4 thick and parchment-like with superficial or deep cracking.

Skin colour

Estimated by inspection when the baby is quiet.

0 dark red
1 uniformly pink
2 pale pink, though the colour may vary over different parts of the body; some parts may be very pale
3 pale; nowhere really pink except on the ears, lips, palms and soles.

Breast size

Measured by picking up the breast tissue between finger and thumb.

0 no breast tissue palpable
1 breast tissue palpable on one or both sides, neither being more than 0.5 cm in diameter

2 breast tissue palpable on both sides, one or both being 0.5 – 1 cm in diameter
3 breast tissue palpable on both sides, one or both being more than 1 cm in diameter.

Ear firmness

Tested by palpation and folding of the upper pinna.

0 pinna feels soft and is easily folded into bizarre positions without springing back into position spontaneously
1 pinna feels soft along the edge and is easily folded but returns slowly to the correct position spontaneously
2 cartilage can be felt to the edge of the pinna though it is thin in places and the pinna springs back readily after being folded
3 pinna firm with definite cartilage extending to the periphery, and springs back immediately into position after being folded.

Table 13.5

Score	*Gestational age (weeks)*	*Score*	*Gestational age (weeks)*
1	27	7	38½
2	30	8	39½
3	33	9	40
4	34½	10	41
5	36	11	41½
6	37	12	42

(Reproduced with kind permission of authors and publishers, from Parkin, J M, Hey, E N, Clowes J S, (1976), Archives of Disease in Childhood, **51**, 259.)

UMBILICAL VEIN CATHETERISATION

General

1. The umbilical vein can usually be catheterised without difficulty up to the 4th day of life. The normal arrangement of vessels is as in Figure 13.10 but is often disturbed by twisting of the cord. The vein is larger and thin-walled, and unless full of clot appears on cross-section as an irregular slit. The arteries are smaller, but have thicker pale-coloured walls; they maintain their shape and usually stand out from the cut surface looking like bits of vermicelli.

2. When possible use a peripheral vein in preference to the umbilical vein, which carries higher risks from infection and thrombosis.

3. When a baby is born who might need catheterisation (e.g. any pre-term or asphyxiated baby) ensure that the cord is cut long so as to leave at least 2 cm clear of the skin.

4. Never leave a catheter unconnected; this can lead to exsanguination or air embolism.

5. Leave catheter in for the least time possible and never for more than 36 hours. Watch carefully for signs of infection, both umbilical and systemic.

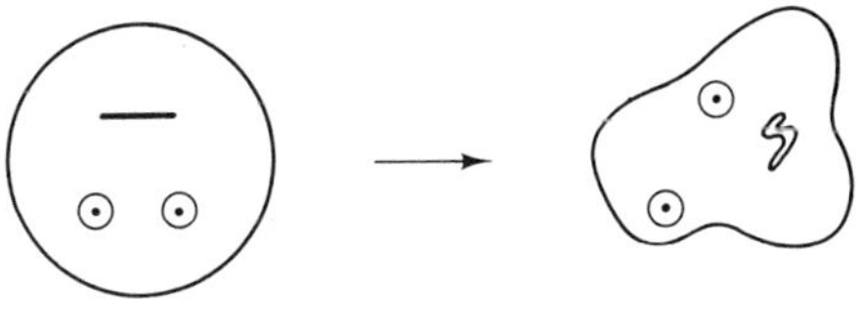

Fig 13.10 Umbilical vessels.

Method

1. Make sure you have the following equipment ready:

Cleansing fluid
Scalpel blade
Blunt-ended catheter with side holes (8 French gauge)
Tape (for securing umbilical stump)
Mosquito forceps
Scissors
Antibiotic spray
Sterile towel (preferably with a hole in middle)
Sterile gauze
Small syringe
Dissecting forceps
Needle with a bent tip as a retractor - see Fig. 13.11
Silk stitch (with needle)
Plaster strapping

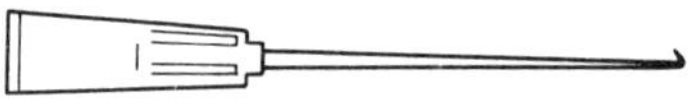

Fig 13.11 Retractor improvised from needle.

2. Ensure that baby is

(i) adequately warmed
(ii) adequately oxygenated
(iii) well restrained.

3. Observe meticulous sterile technique throughout, wearing gown, gloves and mask. Clean abdomen thoroughly, including the umbilical stump, and cover with sterile towel.

4. Tie tape round base of stump so that it can at once be pulled tight in case of unexpected bleeding.

5. With scalpel cut transversely through stump just below any clip or tie that has been previously applied. Carefully clean stump again, and steady it by holding with gauze.

6. Identify vein, steady it with improvised retractor, and extract clot from lumen.

7. Attach syringe to catheter, and holding other end with

forceps inset it into vein aiming towards the heart. It should slide in easily. If it does not you may be making a false passage.

8. If catheter will not go in readily, cut through stump a little lower and try again.

9. Push catheter in until blood flows readily back into syringe. Do not insert too far – you may traverse ductus venosus and enter heart.

10. Take any blood samples that are needed, then quickly connect i.v. infusion and clear catheter of blood to avoid clotting.

11. Tie catheter in position with silk (umbilical stump will usually hold a stitch). Spray stump and surrounding skin with antibiotic spray and secure catheter to abdomen with strapping.

12. When removing the catheter

(i) apply slight suction during withdrawal so that any clot adheres
(ii) tie off vessel with silk
(iii) send tip of catheter for culture.

Appendix: Useful data

AVERAGE WEIGHTS AND BODY SURFACE AREAS

Age	*Weight* *kilos*	*pounds*	*Surface area square metres*
Birth	3.5	7.8	0.21
3 months	5.5	12.1	0.28
6 months	7.5	17	0.35
9 months	9.0	20	0.40
12 months	9.9	22	0.43
18 months	11.3	25	0.48
2 years	12.4	27	0.53
3 years	14.5	32	0.60
4 years	15.5	34	0.68
5 years	18.5	41	0.73
6 years	20.5	44	0.80
7 years	23.0	51	0.87
8 years	25.0	55	0.93
9 years	27.8	61	1.00
10 years	30.5	67	1.08
11 years	34.5	76	1.18
12 years	39.0	86	1.27
13 years	44.5	98	1.39
14 years	50.0	110	1.50
15 years	54.5	120	1.59
16 years	58.0	128	1.65

Weights are medians for children of both sexes, taken with the kind permission of authors and publisher from Tanner J. M. Whitehouse R. H. and Takaishi M. (1966) *Arch. Dis. Child.* **41**, 454. Surface areas are calculated from the same authors' data.

DAILY NEEDS OF FLUID, CALORIES AND ELECTROLYTES

The following should be used as a rough guide only and should be modified to individual situations.

Weight	*Fluid*	*Calories*	Na^+	K^+
kg	ml/kg/day	cal/kg/day	mmol/kg/day	
< 10	120	100	3	3
10-20	100	100	2.5	2.5
> 20	75	75	2.0	2.0

Neonates

Day of life	*Fluid*	
	ml/kg/day	
1	50	(increase initial amounts for a light-for-dates baby) — days 1–2
2	90	
3	120	
4	150	

NORMAL BIOCHEMICAL VALUES FOR BLOOD

	SI units	*'Old units'*	*Conversion*
	mmol/l (unless stated otherwise)	mg/100 ml	SI → mg/100 ml
Bicarbonate	20 - 28		
infants	18 - 23		
Bilirubin	< 14μmol/l	< 0.8	÷ 17
neonates	see p. 000		
Calcium	2.2 - 2.65	8.8 - 10.6	× 4
Creatinine	50 - 140μmol/l	0.6 - 1.6	÷ 90
Glucose	3.3 - 5.6	60 - 100	× 18
neonates	1.0 - 4.1	18 - 73	
Magnesium	0.49 - 0.74	1.2 - 1.8	× 2.4
Potassium	3.5 - 5.0		
infants	4.3 - 6.0		
Sodium	135 - 145		
infants	130 - 140		
Urea	3 - 7	18 - 42	× 6

These values may vary in different laboratories.

NORMAL VALUES FOR CEREBROSPINAL FLUID

Age	*r.b.c.*	*Lymphocytes*	*Protein*	*Glucose*
	per mm^3	per mm^3	gm/l	mmol/l
< 2 weeks	0 - 500	0 - 15	0.3 - 2.0	1.0 - 4
2 - 52 weeks	0	0 - 10	0.2 - 0.6	2.2 - 5
> 1 year	0	0 - 5	0.15 - 0.4	2.2 - 5

CSF glucose is normally c. 1 mmol/l lower than blood glucose, with which it fluctuates.

NORMAL VALUES FOR HAEMOGLOBIN

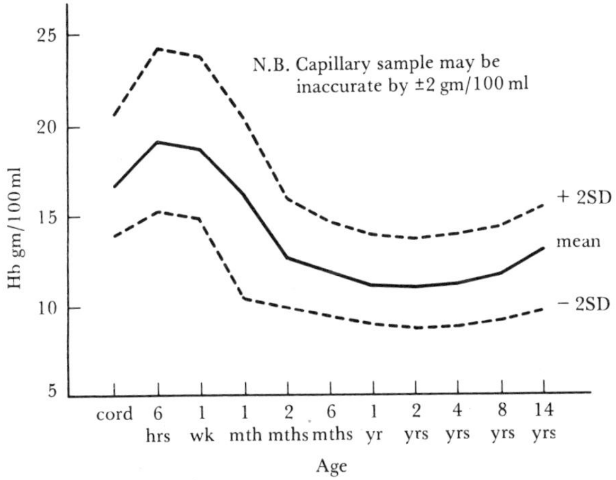

NORMAL VALUES FOR WHITE CELL COUNT

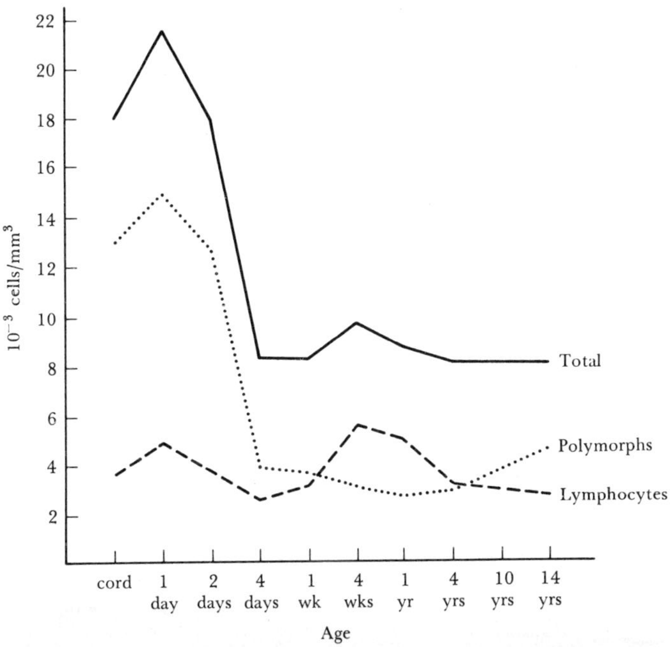

NORMAL ARTERIAL BLOOD GASES AND pH

	kPa	*mm Hg*	*Conversion kPa → mm Hg*
P_{O_2}	11.5 - 13.5 (lower in neonates)	85 - 100	× 7.5
P_{CO_2}	5.3	40	
pH	7.35 - 7.42		

To obtain an *approximate* estimate of arterial values from a mixed venous sample:

P_{CO_2}: subtract 1 kPa (7 mm Hg)
pH: add 0.03
(P_{O_2} cannot be estimated in this way.)

DRUG DOSAGES

NOTES

1. Amounts are in milligrams, unless otherwise stated, and are for each individual dose.

2. Some of the dosages given here can safely be exceeded. *Those which should not be exceeded are given in bold type.*

3. Dosages are suggested for 7 years and for 1 year because a child's surface area is then about a half, and a quarter of an adult's respectively. Adjust dosages for ages in between, and for infants work out dosages per kg.

4. In neonates, especially when pre-term, dosages per kg should be reduced to allow for immature metabolism. Drugs which are contra-indicated or not normally used in neonates are marked *nn.*

5. Routes of administration are denoted as follows:

o oral
m intramuscular
v intravenous
n nebulised
r rectal

Antimicrobials

	Route	Infant	1 yr	7 yrs	Adult	Frequency
Ampicillin	omv	12/kg	125	250	500	6 hrly
Carbenicillin	mv	50/kg	500	1000	2000	6 hrly
Cephaloridine	m	12/kg	125	250	500	8 hrly
Chloramphenicol	omv	**12/kg**	**125**	250	500	6 hrly
Cloxacillin	mv	12/kg	125	250	500	6 hrly
Cotrimoxazole	ov	**4/kg**	40	80	160	12 hrly
Flucloxacillin	o	12/kg	125	250	500	6 hrly
Gentamicin	mv	**2/kg (3/kg in neonates)**	**2/kg**	**2/kg**	**2/kg**	8 hrly
Metronidazole	o	7.5/kg	150	300	600	8 hrly
	v	7.5/kg	7.5/kg	7.5/kg	7.5/kg	8 hrly
Penicillin (benzyl)	mv	15/kg	150	300	600 (=1 megaunit)	6-12 hrly
Penicillin (phenoxymethyl)	o	12/kg	125	250	500	6 hrly
Sulphadimidine	omv	nn	7.5/kg	250	500	6 hrly
Meningitis with unknown organism						
Benzyl penicillin	v	25/kg	3 hrly × 8	then	25/kg	6 hrly
Sulphadimidine	v	**100/kg**	6 hrly × 4	then	**50/kg**	6 hrly
Chloramphenicol	v	**25/kg**	6 hrly × 4	then	**12.5/kg**	6 hrly
Septicaemia with unknown organism						
Benzyl penicillin	v	25/kg	3 hrly × 8	then	25/kg	6 hrly
Gentamicin	v	**3/kg**	8 hrly × 3	then	**2/kg**	8 hrly
				(continue **3/kg** in neonates)		

Note

i.v. boluses of antimicrobials are more effective than infusions, but
(1) observe maker's instructions for dilution and rate of injection,
(2) do not mix two drugs in syringe,
(3) high concentrations of some drugs cause phlebitis.

Other Drugs

	Route	*Infant*	*1 yr*	*7 yrs*	*Adult*	*Frequency*
Aminophylline	v					
loading dose		**6/kg**	**4/kg**	**4/kg**	**4/kg**	× 1 **slowly** (> 5 mins)
infusion		**5/kg/day**	**0.75/kg/hr**	**0.75/kg/hr**	**0.75/kg/hr**	infuse for as long as necessary
Atropine	omv	**0.015/kg**	**0.015/kg**	**0.3**	**0.6**	× 1
Chlorpheniramine	omv	0.25/kg	2.5	5	10	up to 6 hrly
Codeine phosphate	o	nn	15	30	60	up to 4 hrly
Desferrioxamine	omv	nn	see p. 88			
Dexamethasone	omv	nn	2.5	5	10	6 hrly
Diazepam	omr	0.4/kg	0.4/kg	0.4/kg	0.4/kg	up to 6 hrly
	v	**0.2/kg**	**0.2/kg**	**0.2/kg**	**0.2/kg**	up to × 3
			(check respiration between each dose)			
Digoxin	om					
loading dose		**0.03/kg**	**0.03/kg**	**0.5**	**1.0**	× 1 then
		0.01/kg	**0.01/kg**	**0.25**	**0.5**	8 hrly × 2
maintenance		**0.006/kg**	**0.006/kg**	**0.125**	**0.25**	12 hrly
		(individual variation in requirements, so watch for toxicity)				
Frusemide	omv	2/kg	2/kg	2/kg	2/kg	prn
Glucagon	mv	nn	0.25	0.5	1	× 1
Hydrocortisone	mv	25-50	50-100	100	200	prn
Insulin		see p. 70				
Lignocaine (for dysrhythmia)	v	**1/kg**	**1/kg**	**1/kg**	**1/kg**	up to × 4
Mannitol	v	nn	2g/kg	2g/kg	2g/kg	infuse over 60 mins 20% solution
Metoclopramide	omv	0.1/kg	2.5	5	10	up to 6 hrly
Morphine	m	**0.2/kg**	**0.2/kg**	**0.2/kg**	**0.2/kg**	up to 3 hrly
	v	**0.1/kg**	**0.1/kg**	**0.1/kg**	**0.1/kg**	up to 3 hrly
Naloxone	mv	0.1/kg (m) 0.02/kg (v)	0.1	0.4	0.8	4 hrly prn
Paracetamol	or	120	250	500	1000	up to 3 hrly
Paraldehyde	mr	0.1/kg	0.1/kg	0.1/kg	0.1/kg	× 1
Pentazocine	m	nn	1/kg	1/kg	1/kg	up to 3 hrly
	v	nn	0.5/kg	0.5/kg	0.5/kg	
Phenobarbitone	om					
loading dose		**6/kg**	**30**	**60**	**120**	× 1
maintenance		**2.5/kg**	**15**	**30**	**60**	12 hrly
Phenoxybenzamine	v	nn	**1/kg**	**1/kg**	**1/kg**	× 1
Phenytoin (for dysrhythmia)	v	4/kg	4/kg	4/kg	4/kg	up to × 2
Prednisolone	o	0.5/kg	5-10	10-20	15-30	6 hrly
Prochlorperazine	omv	0.125/kg	2.5	5	10	up to 8 hrly
Propranolol	v	**0.01/kg**	**0.01/kg**	**0.01/kg**	**0.01/kg**	repeat up to × 4 cautiously
Salbutamol	o	nn	0.15/kg	4	4-8	6 hrly
	m	nn	0.02/kg	0.02/kg	0.02/kg	6 hrly
	v					
loading dose		nn	**0.004/kg**	**0.004/kg**	**0.004/kg**	× 1 slowly

Other Drugs

	Route	*Infant*	*1 yr*	*7 yrs*	*Adult*	*Frequency*
infusion		nn	**0.24/kg/hr**	**0.24/kg/hr**	**0.24/kg/hr**	infuse for as long as necessary
	n	nn	**0.5 ml**	**1.0 ml**	**1.5 ml**	3 hrly 0.5 % solution
Trimeprazine	om	nn	2-4/kg	2-4/kg	2-4/kg	up to 6 hrly

Index